MW01225332

Better Sex

A Step- by-Step Guide for Beginners to Improve Your Sex Life with Incredible Sex Positions for Couples, and Tips to Explore Your Fantasies and Boost Your Sexual Energy.

Evelyn Jaymes

Table of Contents

Introduction

Who wouldn't want a better sex life if they could? Ask any couple and they would answer with a resounding *YES.* Fuller, richer, and more intensely pleasurable than anything they have ever felt is one of the most rewarding sexual experiences a couple could have together. Almost every couple wants better sex, even if the sex you're having is already good, you wouldn't hesitate at the chance to *make it even better.*

What constitutes better sex, anyway? Lasting longer in bed. Varied positions. Frequent wild and crazy sex. Passion. Chemistry. Compatibility. All these factors and more come together in a culminating, explosive, mind-blowing sexual experience. Everything that you're about to learn in this book is going to help you discover your body (and that of your partner) in the most intimate way. Even if you don't have a significant other at the moment, you could still benefit from the information between these pages. Use it to enhance your sexual knowledge, so the next time you're in bed with someone, you'll knock their socks off when you know what you're doing and why.

Great sex has the power to lift your spirits and make you feel happier. Similarly, bad sex leads to frustration and dissatisfaction. That is why you're here right now. Reading this. You want to enhance the sexual pleasure you and your lover share, and this book is designed to help you do just that. Amazing sex may mean different things to different people, but upskilling your sexual knowledge and venturing beyond your comfort zone is already a step in the right direction.

There are plenty of books on this subject on the market, thanks again for choosing this one! Every effort was made to ensure it is full of as much useful information as possible. Please enjoy!

Chapter 1: How Women Think About Sex and What They Really Want

Unrealistic expectations. Two words that are the quickest way to kill any chance of having mind-blowing sex. Expectations and a lack of communication are problems many couples deal with. The trouble is men and women don't communicate nearly as much as they should about what they *want and need* when it comes to sex. They're okay talking about all the other aspects of their relationship, but with sex, it's different. Many couples often just "do it" without talking about it. They let it happen naturally and go with the flow of the moment, but this approach is exactly what could be ruining the sexual experience for both of you.

Building up these expectations but not expressing them out loud is going to eventually wreak havoc in your relationship, especially if you're in a long-term one. These unrealistic expectations are stopping you from achieving the great sex life you're meant to be having, and it's time to bring that to a halt. Things would certainly be a lot simpler if men and women could understand each other perfectly in bed. Before we begin diving into the details over the next few chapters about how to have better sex, let's begin the first two chapters by taking a closer look at what women and men really want and the way they think about sex.

The Sexual Woman

Most couples are curious about what their partners think of when they're in bed together. They'll be curious, but either to shy or self-conscious to ask out loud. For many women, sex is the deepest expression of love and the connection that they have with their partners. It's true, women don't orgasm as quickly as men do, but *when she does,* it is one of the most powerful, incredible forces that she feels within her. A woman's capacity for pleasure is so great that she's capable of multiple orgasms with the right lover.

One of the few things men and women share is the pressure that they face. The types of sexual pressure they experience might differ, but it is still stressful nonetheless. Women have to deal with pressures of meeting their partner's expectations. Sometimes the pressures they face are the ones they inflict of themselves too, like the expectation that they need to be shaved or waxed or wear sexy lingerie to attract their partners. Not all of these pressures apply to every woman, but some of the common unfair expectations that cause pressure include:

- The expectation that they should orgasm from penetration alone.
- The expectation of orgasming as quickly as men do.
- The expectation that she has no choice but to return the favor if the man goes down on her.
- The mistaken belief that they can get right down to business without the need for foreplay (we can blame bad porn movies and unrealistic

portrayals of romance in the media for that one).

- The misconception that it's a purely physical experience for them too.

The Way She Sees It

A woman's brain works a mile a minute. She's busy and on-the-go, sometimes rarely giving herself a moment to breathe. The way she lives her life has a lot to do with the way that she sees sex and expresses her sexuality. In general, women tend to express their sexuality differently from their male counterparts in the following ways:

- **It Begins In Her Mind** - She may not physically crave it as much as her lover does, but a woman *does* long for sex. She just has a very different way of showing it. Among the main reasons why women differ from men in this department has a lot to do with hormones, mainly the lower levels of testosterone that a woman has in her body. For the woman, sex begins in her mind. When she imagines herself together with her lover, fantasizing about the hot sex they have together, that's what gets her engines going.

- **The Longing to Be Desired -** When a woman feels desired, that's when the sexual goddess within her comes alive. Meredith Chivers, a sex researcher, claims feeling desired *IS the orgasm.* This depends on the woman, of course, since some tend to be a lot more visually stimulated than others. But when she sees an attractive man, the thought that will be running through her mind is whether he finds her sexually attractive or not. When she knows with certainty that the man craves her body and is hungry for her in that way, her imagination (sex begins in the mind after all) starts to run wild. The more she fantasizes about the two of them being together, the more aroused she starts to get as her brain begins to generate one sexy image and fantasy after another.

- **It's Complicated** - Well, sexually anyway. While most women do want sex and even love doing it with their partner, there's a lot of other factors that come into play that could easily derail her desire. Tiredness is the most common factor, what with the busy and hectic lives that we lead. Other factors could include anything from anger, resentment, the trauma of any past experiences, physiological troubles that include physical pain. Even menopause affects their libido to a certain extent. Women are prone to multi-tasking, and it's hard for her to put her brain on pause and come to bed willingly when she's got a lot of other thoughts running in her mind.

- **It Depends on the Context** - Nearly all men begin their first foray into the sexual world through masturbation. For a woman, a large portion of their sexual lives begins with their very first hook-up or serious relationship. The first time many women are touched intimately is when they're with a partner. Women want to feel the pleasure of being touched by their lover in such an intimate manner, and this is a vulnerability in its rawest form. She may be reluctant to open her heart to her partner because she's afraid of getting hurt, and this might cause her to withdraw physically from her significant other. Women *need to feel safe* on an emotional level, and this point cannot be emphasized enough. Therefore, it is important that she works together with her lover to co-create a context where she feels safe enough to let her defenses down and willing to expose her vulnerability.

- **Love Is an Aspect of It -** Sex, to a woman, is part of the overall package. It is not the defining factor of a relationship. It is *part* of it. Having sex, being together as a couple, living together, sharing laughs together, celebrating special moments, managing responsibilities as a team, giving and receiving love and affection. It all comes together for her. Sex is one of the many ways she expresses her love for her partner.

What She Thinks About It & What She Wants from You

The thing that a lot of men fail to understand is that a woman *does not* need to orgasm for the sex to be satisfying. Not that she would say no to a climax, of course, but to her, it is the intimate bond and connection that is more fulfilling than curling her toes and screaming her lover's name. Women are prone to faking orgasms because they don't want their partners to feel bad, which is the problem a lot of men tend to have in the bedroom. When they can't make their partner orgasm, they believe they have failed or that they may be terrible in bed.

If only we could read each other's minds. Sex would be a lot happier and less anxiety-ridden.

Unfortunately, we can't, but that's why you're here and why you're reading this book. To find out what women and men *really* think about sex. Let's begin with what women think and what she wants from her lover:

- **Don't Exaggerate -** It's always flattering to be told how beautiful or sexy you are, but one mistake a man might make is when he tries to go overboard with the compliments. Women want to be complimented, but complimented *honestly.* There's no need to tell her that she looks like Heidi Klum in bed when she knows that's far from the truth. Exaggeration only makes the compliments sound insincere, and it's killing her libido. Instead, what she wants is to hear compliments that come from the heart. It does not always have to be focused on looks either. Compliment her when she's gone out of her way to do something for you, compliment the way she takes care of you and makes you feel loved. Tell her that you love her or how beautiful she looks when she's wearing something flattering.

- **Being Objectified Is Not Always A Bad Thing -** Not all women are prudes, and there can be something incredibly sexy about being overpowered or objectified every now and then by her lover. As long as it is kept only in the bedroom, of course. Dirty talk is a turn on for some women. Both partners need to be on the same page about this, though, before you begin. If you don't mind being objectified every now and then by your man and it is feeding into a secret fantasy, let him know you're okay with it. He might be just as keen to give it a go.

- **Nice and Slow -** When a man is nice and slow, taking his time worshipping every inch of her body instead of rushing to get down to business, it strokes her ego and reinforces how much her lover enjoys her body. Women want to be touched sensually and kissed passionately, and they enjoy a healthy mix of slow and rough passion. It's not a hard and fast rule, though, it would depend on the woman's preference and what she feels like at the time. There may be times when her hormones are so riled up that she'll be more than happy for you to rip her clothes off and start pounding her hard.

- **Hear Your Moan -** Some women love hearing their partner's vocally express how good it feels to be making love. Men are not the only ones who get turned on by a woman who moans his name in the heat of passion. When a man is expressive, grunting, swearing, or even moaning every now and then, it lets her know that he is enjoying this as much as she is.

- **Being Hands-On Is Good -** Women love a man who knows what to do with his hands. Since a lot of women have a hard time achieving an orgasm from penetration alone, a partner who knows how to work some magic with his fingers is exactly what she needs to get her off. Tease her nipples, massage her breasts sensually when you kiss her passionately, stimulate her clit with your fingers when you're having sex, and she'll be begging you for more.

- **A Little Kink Can Be a Good Thing -** Sex should be exciting and just as passionate as it was the day you first started. Switching things up every now and then adds variety. Not every woman wants to stick to plain, old vanilla sex alone. That can quickly become monotonous, and surprisingly a lot of women are more open to the idea of rough, kinky sex if both partners are on the same page about it. Try new positions, surprise her with new moves, do it in places other than the bedroom. Experiment and be adventurous about it.

We Need to Talk About It

As important as it is to be satisfied in bed, it is even more important to talk about sexual health for both men and women. A woman's sexual health encompasses physical and emotional aspects, both of which are important to the state of her wellbeing. When she experiences a sex life that is fulfilling, she's less stressed, and the quality of her sleep is better. Unlike men, a woman's physical desire for sex does not motivate or dictate her sexual activity. Women are stimulated by various motivators. What gets one woman aroused might do nothing for someone else.

Women over the age of 40 and those who have undergone menopause have different motivators when it comes to sex. Instead of being driven by hormones, it is now the feeling of intimacy and closeness that she has with her partner that arouses her the most. It's hard to define what sexual satisfaction is for women since not everyone experiences the same thing. It is not easy for a lot of couples to talk about their sexual needs. Women complain that men don't communicate enough, even worse when it comes to sexual matters. Yet, communication is the one thing you need to start doing for a sex life that is happier, healthier, and filled with greater levels of satisfaction between the sheets.

Learning to talk about your sexual health, experiences, any thoughts or expectations you may or may not have brings you closer together as a couple. Since it's not an easy subject to bring up out of the blue, here's what you can do to ease into the process:

- **Admit What You Feel** - Maybe you feel anxious, shy, nervous, scared of having of heart broke, worried you're going to disappoint your partner in bed. It's okay to experience these thoughts and emotions, they're perfectly normal, and more importantly, it's okay to talk about them to your partner. Bring up any concerns you have and be honest about it. Explain your reasons behind the way you feel or what you think, help your partner understand where you're coming from. Ask them for what you need to feel better about the whole thing. You're in this together, and sex is a two-way street. It takes two people working together to make magic happen.

- **Put It on A Timer -** If the very idea of talking openly about sex with your partner makes you feel overwhelmed or anxious, what might help is to set the conversation on a time limit. Knowing that the conversation is not going to last for long makes you feel better on a psychological level and this way, you know you're not forcing yourself to push past your comfort zone. Women are emotional and that is a fact, and it is important that these emotions be well-regulated and taken care of instead of being dismissed like they don't mean anything. Your emotions matter and your partner should understand and respect this.

- **Make Sex Conversations A Regular Thing -** Once you've opened this can of worms (so to speak), you want to try and make this a regular routine if you can. The more you learn to talk about your sex life, expectations, sexual health, and what you need from your partner, the conversations start to get easier over time. Eventually, you'll be comfortable enough to openly ask for what you need from your man to feel satisfied without feeling shy or embarrassed about it.

What to Do When Your Sexual Needs Are Different

Men and women are as different as night and day. Yet, this is a fact that we forget, and the main reason why we start to worry and fret when our partner does not react the way we expect them too.

Having sexual needs that are different may sometimes contribute to feelings of rejection, isolation, resentment, or isolation. We forget to consider the fact that maybe our partner may not feel the same way we do. This only goes to show how important it is for couples to communicate and openly talk about *every* aspect of their sex life. Communication is the only way to deal with the gap in your needs. Talking about it is the only way to explore and discuss other options and to work on finding a solution that will leave everyone feeling happy.

Chapter 2: How Men Think About Sex and What They Really Want

Men think about sex *all the time.* Well, that's the stereotypical perception anyway. How much truth is there to that statement, though? Do they think about sex *that* much? The stereotype seems a little excessive, and several researchers have set out to prove exactly how often men have sex on their minds. One study by *The Journal of Sex Research* did confirm that men think a lot more about sex than their female counterparts do. About 19 times a day, on average, to be exact, whereas women think about sex maybe 10 times a day.

Some studies even claim men think about sex every seven seconds, and if those statistics are to be believed, that would mean that men think about sex 514 times within an hour or 7,200 times approximately throughout his waking hours. That seems like an awful lot of times. You have to wonder how they get anything done in that state. Interestingly enough, there have been scientific attempts by psychologists to measure thoughts in a technique referred to as experience sampling.

A research team from Ohio State University attempted to carry out this experiment by giving their test subjects "clickers." The 283 college students partaking in the study were allocated into three groups. They were asked to record and press their clickers each time they thought about sex, food, and sleep. The results of the study revealed that the average male in this study thought about sex approximately 19 times a day while the average woman thought about it 10 times per day. The results also indicated that men thought a lot more about food and sleep than women did, which might imply that men had a higher tendency to give in to their indulgent impulses. The interesting outcome of the study was the revelation about the large variation in the number of thoughts the participants recorded. Some respondents only thought about sex once a day while the top responded reported an astounding 388 clicks, which suggested they had a sexual thought at least every two minutes.

What Does Sex Mean to Him?

It's no secret that men view sex from an entirely different perspective. A common misconception is that men are into sex only for their benefit and pleasure. That's not always the case (depending on the man, of course). If you let them, most men want to help their lovers achieve orgasm and enjoy sex as much as they do. It's easy to assume that all men are the same, but that's an unfair stereotype.

While every man is different, some of the common themes about a man's general perception of sex include the following:

- **It's A Physical Thing** - For men, the desire for sex is physical, and given the high levels of testosterone in their bodies, it is easy to see why. This hormone is responsible for driving them to express their sexual needs. When an erection springs forth at even the slightest hint of provocation in younger men, that's the testosterone at play. Men are visual creatures, and the mere sight of his partner coming out of the shower naked or getting dressed is enough to cause a physical reaction in his body.

- **They Are *Hungry* for It -** It's not an exaggeration to say men crave sex the way anyone would crave for food when they are hungry. There's a strong physical need within them to have this craving fulfilled. A day wouldn't be complete if you didn't have your meals, and that's what a man feels like about sex. If they could have it every day, they would love to. Sex quite literally satisfies their carnal appetite.

- **It's Energetic -** All those raging hormones in his body are infusing him with energy. The prospect of having sex is exciting to him, and it is what keeps him going throughout the day, pushing through an otherwise mundane routine to get the day over with if he knows his partner is waiting for him at home ready to fulfill is lustful fantasies. To a man, especially a young man, a sexual counter is a thrilling new adventure. His body thrives on the pleasure he derives from sex and it will never be enough, even if he had sex every day. Since a man's orgasm is a lot easier to achieve than a woman's, every position, rhythm, role-play, smile, image, innuendo, shapely body and fantasy is an opportunity for sexual gratification. Whether he's fantasizing about it or if it's happening for real, the excitement derived from any sexual-related experience is enough to cause a spike in his brainwaves.

- **It's How He Shows/Gives Love Too -** This is one of the few things men and women have in common in this department. With the right lover, sex is how a man shows his love. He loves knowing that he could satisfy his lover in bed and make her beg for more. He loves being the one who is responsible for the pleasure that they felt together when they were making love. In his heart, a man wants his lover to feel as much exquisite pleasure as he does and he's willing to put in the work if it means a chance to bring her to a climax.

- **When It's Love, It's Home -** There's no experience quite like making passionate love to someone you're in love with. For a man, the sexual release is akin to the feeling of coming home. No matter what kind of day you've had, there's no place like home to make it all better, and sex with someone he loves is the embodiment of those emotions. Lovemaking is the way a man and a woman come together to form a deep, meaningful attachment built on love and trust. Women crave for the emotional connection to feel safe. For men, it is the sexual connection they have with their lovers that gives them that same sense of security.

What He Thinks About It

It is a shame that we're programmed to believe talking about sex is taboo or embarrassing. Couples could have significantly more satisfying relationships if only they learned to communicate about what they wanted (or didn't want) in bed. Men are just as uncomfortable talking about the subject as women are. They may be confident enough doing the deed, but expressing what they want from you sexually is a different matter altogether. Partners should be curious and inquisitive about what turns each other on. What does he want in bed? What can a woman do to increase the intensity of the pleasure he feels? For that to happen, she needs to *know what he wants* otherwise, it's going to be next to impossible for the emotional and physical intimacy to take place. There can be no deep and meaningful emotional connection without communication.

Ever wondered what men *really think* about sex and what they want from their lovers? Let's find out:

- **The Nuance of Sexiness -** The way she flirts with her eyes, the way her hips move when she talks, the way she talks, the way she comes alive and gets excited when her favorite song is on the radio. All those little details add up and contribute to what men find sexy about their lover.

- **The Novelty of Hotness Doesn't Last -** Being hot may be great in the beginning, since men are visual by nature, but eventually, the novelty starts to wear off. Being hot doesn't necessarily mean the sexual chemistry is great. Looks don't last forever, and there's more to great lovemaking than the way a woman looks or how her body feels. Men are attracted to a woman's physical appearance at first, no doubt, but at the end of the day, it's her personality and the kind of woman she is that will decide how great they are in bed together.

- **The Need to Objectify Is Purely Sexual -** They may support feminism and strong female empowerment, but within the sexual context, the need to objectify you at times is primal. Men are enraptured by the way her body moves, how soft her skin is, and addicted to the corves of her body. They respect their lovers, but they still want them to be a goddess in bed.

- **Their Penis Is Their Manhood -** There is something incredibly seductive about a woman who knows how to worship her man's penis. A man sees his penis as an extension of his manhood, and when a woman shows equal excitement for it, his existing attraction to her immediately skyrockets up a few more notches. Men want their penises to be worshipped by their lovers the same way he worships her vagina and all its glory when he goes down on her.

- **A Lot of Kinky Thoughts Happen -** Sometimes, the sexual thoughts men have might shock their lovers. Men watch a lot of porn. *A lot of porn* and they are obsessed with the power of female sexuality. They will think about doing the dirtiest, nastiest, kinkiest thing to their partners from time to time.

- **They Care About Her Orgasms -** It empowers their masculinity when they know they could make their partners orgasm in bed and call out their name in pleasure. It makes them feel like a man when they know they've managed to make their partners come. Even better when he's able to give her multiple orgasms. Her screams of pleasure are the confidence to boost his needs for his sexual prowess.

- **They Want a Lot of Sex -** Men want it more than women do, although by now this probably comes as no surprise. A *Men's Health* survey that involved 6,700 participants (men and women) revealed that one-third of the women who were surveyed were having sex at least two, if not three, times a week. 71% of the women surveyed said they were "satisfied" or "thrilled" when asked about their sex lives. The men in the survey were having sex about the same number of times, but only 51% of the respondents said they were "thrilled" or "satisfied" when asked the same question. The possible reasons attributed to this lack of enthusiasm by the male respondents include that they wanted more sex and they were not getting it.

- **They Want Affection Too** - Women are not the only ones who want to feel loved and shown affection by their lovers. Men want the same thing too, although they're probably less vocal about it. Men want to kiss, touch, cuddle, and have sweet nothings whispered in their ears during sex too. They want to be told what a turn-on they are, to know they're partners find them irresistible too. Research indicates that men and women mutually benefit from affectionate and romantic behaviors, and this was one of the traits both sexes found appealing about their significant other.

- **They Can Be as Sexually Committed As You Are -** Not every man is only interested in casual sex. Research by the *National Survey of Sexual Health and Behavior* discovered that men were happier and found sex more enjoyable and fulfilling when they were in a committed relationship. The same research revealed that men in a committed relationship experienced greater orgasms; they were more aroused and experienced fewer issues like erectile dysfunction, for example.

What Men Want as They Grow Older

As they mature, a man's needs and wants have changed. They're no longer the hormonally-charged teenagers eager to hop into bed at a moment's notice. As they mature, what a man wants in bed changes from what he wanted when he was in his 20s or 30s. By the time he's hit the mid-point of his life, he's established what works for him sexually and they want a lover who understands their needs as well as her own.

He's older, he's wiser, and he's got a bit more experience under his belt. He knows what he wants and what he needs to feel good and now he's looking for a partner he can share that with. Men in their mid-life want a lover who is:

- **Confident** - Gone are the days when you're both young, insecure, and trying to figure out what you want out of life. By this point, a man wants a woman who is comfortable in her own skin and confident about her sexuality. They appreciate a woman who knows what she wants and is not afraid to express herself.

- **Communicative** - Both sexes would have been around the block long enough that communicating what you need shouldn't be an uncomfortable subject any longer. Communication at this age is just as important as it was when they were young and virile. A man can't read your mind, and he's not interested anymore in playing mind games by this stage of life. To him, a woman is at her sexiest when she knows her body and is comfortable enough to tell him how she likes to be pleasured.

- **Spontaneous** - Surprises can any age can keep the excitement alive. Having sex for this many years can make it feel a little mundane, and some spontaneity keeps the anticipation alive. Surprise him with a new position. Try doing it somewhere new or introduce a new toy during foreplay.

- **Easy to Satisfy** - The thrill of a challenge is great when you're young and driven primarily by hormones. However, a man's preference shifts over time. Most men by this age want to know they can easily satisfy their partner, and more importantly, he *wants her to let him know when* she is satisfied. A woman who fakes her orgasms is no longer a turn-on or a novelty. He's no longer interested in a woman who will tell him everything he wants to hear, whether or not it's true. His satisfaction comes from knowing he could satisfy her on every level.

- **Willing to Take It Slow -** The days of ripping each other's clothes off in a hurry to get to the main event are not the focus anymore. By mid-life, both sexes are well aware of the fact that there is more to sex than the physical aspect alone. Slowing things down, taking time to savor each other's bodies as you work your way up to the grand finale is the most pleasurable aspect of sex now. Intimate touching, kissing, cuddling, masturbation, these elements still need to be present if the man and his partner are going to be satisfied.

- **His Equal -** He wants a lover, not a child or a mother. He appreciates the loving and caring things that you do for him, but between the sheets, he wants intimacy, passion, and romance. He wants an equal partner who is passionate, confident, and knows how to show her man some love.

- **A Positive Force -** Men in their mid-life are aware of the fact that they may not be as young and robust in the sack as they were during their prime. They're probably self-conscious about it on some level, which explains the need to know they are still capable of pleasing their partners. They want a woman who is a positive force in bed and knows how to reassure her man he's doing a good job. They want someone who appreciates them. If he makes her feel good, it reinforces his confidence and lets him know that he's still got it in him to make a woman cry out in pleasure. Telling a man that what he's doing feels good is a huge turn on, whether they're younger or older. A woman who is supportive and encouraging will go a lot more his libido than someone who nitpicks and focuses on everything that he could be doing better.

Chapter 3: You Come First

There's nothing like the emotional, happy high that you get from being in a loving, committed relationship. When you're genuinely happy, everything is right with the world, and your lover can do no wrong. The happy glow and the smile on your face can be seen from a mile away. Your family and your friends notice this new positive change about you, now that you have this one special person in your life. You can't believe your good fortune that you've managed to land someone as incredible as your partner.

Is this really happening? Is he/she in love with me? What if they leave me once they realize my flaws?

A healthy and happy relationship that is thriving and going strong can only exist when both partners are comfortable with themselves *and* with each other. A relationship cannot keep going strong for long if it is filled with doubt and insecurity. The very idea of being vulnerable, leaving yourself open to possibly being hurt emotionally – especially by the ones closest to you – is not an idea that many are going to stomach easily. The very first question you would probably be asking yourself is, *why on earth would I want to subject myself to being hurt that way?* That's perfectly understandable. Unless you've already got a boatload of courage buried deep within you, being vulnerable and wearing your heart on your sleeve is going to prove to be a challenge.

Loving Yourself the Most

Trusting someone is something that takes time, but to be able to trust them enough to freely be who you are, you're going to need to open yourself to be vulnerable. What makes this process difficult is that by being completely open and honest in this way, you're leaving the door wide open for the other person to hurt you. For love to blossom, happiness *must* be a priority. There's no exception to this rule.

Couples must love each other despite their flaws, and before you can trust that your partner loves and accepts you for who you are, *you need to accept and love yourself*. If you find it hard to love and respect yourself, how do you expect anyone else to love you the way you deserve?

Confidence is an attractive quality for both men and women for a reason. When you love yourself, you see your true value. You know what your strengths are and why anyone would be lucky to have you as a partner, so you don't question your lover's motives and wonder what on earth they're doing with you when they could probably be with someone better. Loving yourself means you know what you want and what you're not willing to put up with. You're not going to tolerate anything less than you deserve that threatens to take away your happiness. Put your happiness first, and everything else falls into place, including being in a mutually respectful and loving relationship.

The more you love yourself, the less you will rely on your partner to validate your self-worth. Placing your value in the hands of another is how you become insecure and needy in your relationship. You're so worried your partner is going to find someone else that you're not focused enough on trying to strengthen the relationship. Relinquishing control by seeking validation externally is never going to bring any true happiness and insecurity is a chemistry killer. It won't be long before the initial passion that drew you to each other diminishes when not enough time is being spent nurturing the relationship because your partner is too busy having to reassure you that you're worthy of being loved.

When you love yourself, you know what you want. You know what kind of partner you deserve. You know what you want to get out of your relationship. You know where you want to be several years from now and you're not willing to settle for less than the best. Loving yourself is the best thing you can do for your happiness. Long-lasting happiness needs to come from within. When you're happy with yourself and the life you have, finding someone to share that love and happiness with is a bonus, not a necessity. A man and woman should never rely on each other as the main source of happiness. What happens if that source is gone one day? The only person responsible for your happiness is you and it is the only way to ensure that no matter what happens in your life, you're strong enough to bounce back from it. Even if you lose your relationship.

Understanding Your Sexual Pleasures

Ask anyone what kind of sex they want to have, and they'll tell you they want "great sex." Yet, not everyone can define what "great sex" means to them and there's a very good reason for this. *They don't understand their bodies enough.* They don't know the way their body reacts and *why* it reacts the way it does to certain stimuli. They don't know what techniques work best on themselves and their partners. Some might not even be aware of what their erogenous zones are. It's going to be hard to have "great sex" unless you know your body well enough inside at out. So let's get to know your body better:

- **Your Erogenous Zones -** Essentially, these are the areas of your body with lots of nerve endings that get you aroused or excited when they're touched in the right way. The biggest erogenous zones in the body for most people are the vagina, penis, vulva, labia, clitoris, prostate, perineum, anus, and the scrotum. Out of these, it is generally the clitoris and the penis that are the most sensitive zones. Everyone's body is different, and for some, their erogenous zones might their neck, butt, breasts, thighs, feet, mouth, and nipples. To find out which areas excite you the most, you need to experiment until you hit the sweet spot (or your partner does).

- **The Sex Cycle Response -** This describes the way that your body reacts when it is sexually stimulated. This cycle could either happen alone or with your partner. The sex cycle happens in several stages. The first stage is desire, where thinking sexual thoughts begins to arouse and excite you, getting your body primed and ready for sex. The second stage of the cycle is the plateau stage, and you're fully aroused by this point, ready to either have sex or masturbate. The third and final stage of the cycle is the orgasm phase when all that sexual tension that has been building up is finally released and your body convulses with pleasure.

- **Explore Your Body -** It's time to get intimate with yourself if you haven't done that already. Before you can understand what turns you on, you need to give yourself an anatomy lesson. Learn to please your body through self-stimulation and exploration. It's okay to be nervous about this in the beginning, touching yourself intimately in that way may feel strange and unfamiliar at first. Take your time exploring yourself thoroughly, so you know what turns you on and what causes discomfort. Our understanding of our bodies affects your mindset and the more comfortable you are with your body, the easier it will be to succumb to the pleasure when you're with your lover.

- **Understanding Orgasms** - Sexual stimulation doesn't need to happen to experience an orgasm. Most couples would be surprised to know this. There are a few ways to define what an orgasm means. Medical professionals think of it as the physiological change that the body undergoes. Psychologists see it as your body experiencing cognitive and emotional changes. At the moment, there's no overarching description that succinctly depicts what an orgasm means, but what we do know is that it feels *extremely good* when it happens. Orgasms have a few categories too. Multiple orgasms, G-spot orgasms, fantasy orgasms, relaxation orgasms, tension orgasms, and a combination of the different experiences coming together. Which one you experience depends on the context in which it is happening.

Sexuality is a constant state of exploration. Depending on how comfortable you are and how long you've been in a relationship, you'll be curious, pushing your boundaries and exploring just how far you can go. We evolve and grow with time, and so does our sexuality. It's not a permanent state of being. It's a work in progress, one that you must give yourself time to adjust to. Your body is a source of pleasure and it is time you got to know that.

The Way to Better Female Orgasms

Pleasure is different for everyone and you shouldn't believe everything that you watch in porn. Getting an orgasm is a unique experience for each woman and it is still very much an area of mystery for both sexes. Believe it or not, women don't need to climax to be sexually happy and satisfied by their lovers. Too much pressure is placed on women achieving orgasm the way a man does, which is practically at every sexual encounter. Men feel pressured when their partner doesn't orgasm, and it makes him question his capabilities, while women feel pressured enough to fake an orgasm because they don't want to disappoint their partners. This might have something to do with the innate fear we all have about being "rejected" if we fail to live up to the sexual expectations placed upon us. Needless to say, this is going to be an orgasm killer for many women.

Not helping matters is the taboo that has been surrounding the subject of women and self-exploration for a long time. The notion that "good girls" don't touch themselves in that way has made many of us feel uncomfortable and even ashamed of our natural desires. Female sexual pleasure is one of the least talked about subjects, but it is a subject you need to start embracing. Sexual satisfaction can only be achieved (alone or with your partner) when you know *what works for you.*

- Take as much time as you need getting to know your body. Don't be afraid to use your fingers and a couple of toys during your exploration process.

- Explore stimulating and putting pressure on your clitoris and see how you feel.

- Touch your body all over when you're in the shower and explore every inch and hidden crevice in detail. It's an exercise in getting to know your various body parts.

- Wear a blindfold when you masturbate alone and let your other senses come alive to replace the one that has been temporarily taken aware. This heightened sensitivity makes you aware of what stimulation gets you off the most.

- Follow good old-fashioned advice and grab a mirror and look at yourself down there.

- Explore stimulating your clitoris, vagina, vulva and the surrounding area with your fingers or with sex toys if you prefer. Try different strokes, positions, and varying degrees of pressure to see what brings you closer to the big O.

Postponing Your Ejaculation

Nature made is such that women are fortunate enough to experience prolonged orgasms that come in waves. A man's orgasm, on the other hand, is brief but explosive, lasting anywhere from 5-7 seconds at a time. Men would love if this feeling could last longer than a couple of seconds no doubt, but so far, there's no tried and true method to keep the orgasm going for longer. One study reveals that between the age of 18 and 60, at least 30% of men within this age group will prematurely ejaculate at some point. It may not always happen, but when it does, it is characterized as ejaculation happening within a minute of penetration most of the time.

The good news is, there are ways you can delay it. You may not be able to prolong the sensation, but you can prolong the pleasure and delay the orgasm enough so you last longer.

To delay what inevitably is going to happen, a man needs to get as close to the threshold as possible, and then halt. Stop the stimulation, breathe, and relax all the muscles around the lower back and perineum. Wait until the sensation has passed before you begin the stimulation again. It sounds easy enough in theory, but it takes considerable effort, mental and emotional discipline, and a lot of willpower for him to pull himself back from the brink of sexual bliss. The trick to making this technique work is to reach the highest state of excitement right before he is about to ejaculate and then forcibly pull back. By withholding himself from the pleasure, he is opening the door for even greater levels of excitement the next time he is stimulated. Keep the cycling going by reaching high and then pulling back as many times as possible until he can finally take no more. The best way to practice this technique is when you're masturbating alone. Do what you would normally do to self-stimulate, come close, and then pull back. See how many times you can repeat the process until you finally release all that pent up energy and ejaculate with gusto.

Other techniques you could try include:

- **Squeeze It -** To bring your happy ending to a halt, try squeezing the shaft of your penis right before you're about to ejaculate. Give it a good squeeze between your thumb and forefinger, but to the point where it's causing you pain. The act of squeezing it is going to minimize your erection slightly so you can spend more time going at it with your partner.

- **The Diversion -** When you're about to reach your peak, let your mind wander and distract it from the sensation that you feel in your nether regions. Distraction and diversion shift your mind and your body away from the focus of peaking too early.

- **Breathe Deeply -** To successfully mitigate your ejaculation, breathe from your diaphragm when you're making love to your partner. This technique is referred to as "*diaphragm* *breathing"* or *"belly breathing."* When you're about to come, your breathes tend to be shorter, sharp, and shallow which will cause your heart rate to spike. By controlling your breathing with deep, measured, in and out breaths, you're actively regulating the sensations you feel through mindful awareness, allowing you to focus on controlling your ejaculation.

- **Spray It to Delay It -** If all else fails, there's always the option of using topical sprays to help you delay the process. These sprays are applied at least 10-minutes prior to sex and directly on the penis. Spritz it a couple of times, and you'll be ready to go strong for the next 30 minutes or so. Maybe even 60 minutes for some men.

The Man's Secret to Multiple Orgasms

It's not a myth. Women are not the only ones capable of multiple orgasms. The man's secret to doing the same lies in a gland that is no bigger than the size of a walnut. *Your prostate.* When stimulated enough, a man is more than capable of achieving a full-blown orgasm, *even* if he is not fully erect to do it. The only thing is a lot of straight men might find this uncomfortable since to get to the prostate, they or their partners will have to access it through the anus or alternatively, under the perineum area. But once they get past that initial apprehension though, *everything* changes,

A lot of straight men struggle with the idea of letting their partners stimulate their anus. They're even *more* uncomfortable with having to do it themselves. This hang-up has more to do with the mindset than anything else. Enjoying the pleasure of anal stimulation has nothing to do with what your sexual preference may be. It takes a man who is open-minded enough to get past this way of thinking, and if it means you now have access to the secret of multiple orgasms, why not?

If you are attempting this by yourself or with your partner, use a lot of water-based lube to avoid hurting the sensitive tissue around the area. You can either do this by yourself or with your partner. When you're ready, gently slide your lubed-up finger into your anus. Allow your body time to get comfortable with the sensation and then begin to angle your finger towards the direction of your penis. Once you feel slight pressure, that's when you know you've found the right spot. It's going to feel a little like you have to pee before the sensation begins to shift from intense pleasure to oh-my-god orgasmic bliss.

Chapter 4: Approaching Sex

Sex is not the easiest topic to bring up, especially when you're naturally the shy type or when you're starting out with a new partner. When you're shy by nature, even the idea of talking about it out loud is enough to make you want to flee. We've all got bits we're a wee bit insecure or bashful about. Thankfully, there are ways to overcome your shyness, so you don't have to miss out on having a fulfilling sex life.

Unleashing your sexual side in front of another can be terrifying, exciting, and intimidating all rolled into one. Women, in particular, tend to be extremely self-conscious and sometimes insecure about their bodies, which only aggravates the shyness that they feel.

Overcoming Shyness

Shyness on its own is not that big of a problem. Unless it is holding you back from being romantically intimate with your partner. You know you don't want to be alone and you know you love your partner, yet feeling shy about your body and your skills in bed is something you can't quite shake.

Coming out of your shell is going to change your relationship and the way that you connect to your partner in a major way. If the sex is good now, imagine what it is going to be like when you can shed your inhibitions and give yourself over completely to the experience?

- **Make the First Step A Small Step -** As a shy person, rushing headfirst into anything is never the way to go. For one thing, you could react impulsively and say or do something you regret, and if you're already shy, rushing through it is not going to make you feel any better. The first step is to *take a small step,* and this is the easy part. All you need to do here is to acknowledge the way that you feel. Think about what you need to feel comfortable in the bedroom. Soothing music? Scented candles in the background with scents that relax your mind? Eating chocolate? Having a glass of wine before you get to lovemaking? These are easy conversation starters, and what you could do is ask your partner what makes them feel comfortable in bed too.

- **Taking Control -** Feeling self-conscious might have to do with the fact that you know your partner is looking at you. If you're working up the courage towards some bolder, more adventurous sex moves, one technique that might work is to blindfold your partner so he *can't see you*. Eliminating their sense of sight will heighten all the other senses, and now that you know they can't see what you're doing, you start to feel a little more confident and start making moves you might not want to do when someone is watching you.

Alternatively, try making love in positions that require you to turn away from each other if that makes you feel better.

- **A Wheel of Passion -** An activity you could work on if one or both partners are shy about broaching the subject of sex is to create a *Wheel of Passion* together. It's a little brainstorming activity you can do together. Get a blank piece of paper and write *Wheel of Passion* in bold letters at the top. Next, draw a large circle right in the center and divide that circle into 10 segments. It should look like 10 pieces of a pie when you're done. Next, take turns writing down passionate activities inside the wheel and it should be activities that make you feel the most passionate. It could be kissing, sexual massages, quickies, oral sex, self-stimulation, erotic sensual talk, intercourse, anything that you want. Each partner writes down five activities that they need to feel passionate about when making love. Doing this together helps you overcome the shyness knowing you're not doing it alone. Even better when you find your partner may have the same passion activities that you do.

- **Praise Your Partner -** It is important to let your partner know that they're doing a good job. That your shyness has nothing to do with their skills in bed. Your body might feel tense when you find it hard to relax and be yourself, and if your partner doesn't understand the reasons why, they may interpret that as a sign that you think they're terrible, or worse, that you don't want them touching you that way.

- **Engage in Self-Pleasure -** Masturbating is the link you've been looking for to boost your confidence about your sexuality. Despite what we have been programmed to believe, sex is not dirty and touching yourself is not "wrong." To overcome your shyness, you need to give yourself permission to feel pleasure. Why? Because *why not?* Sex is a basic human need, and like every other need, it must be fulfilled.

You need to get comfortable with touching yourself in the most intimate way possible, or you're always going to be hesitant and awkward about letting someone else do it. Your body is a stranger and you need to spend some quality alone time getting to know it better until *you feel better* about your body. Part of the reason you're insecure is that you don't know your body and what you like. Learn to see masturbation as a good thing and get accustomed to the pleasure. Once you let your body acclimatize to how good it feels, your confidence will begin to develop along with once you start craving for those pleasurable sensations.

- **Buy Sex Clothing -** This step is meant for women since men don't generally have or wear a lot of sexy clothing to begin with. If you're ever going to feel confident about your sexuality, you need to *see yourself as a sexual being*. A quick and effective way to do this is to dress the part. Purchase clothing that makes you feel good about yourself when you put it on. Look in the mirror and admire how the lingerie accentuates your curves and how good the soft, silky material feels against your skin. Your body is beautiful the way it is, and it's time to get over those mental hang-ups you have about the way you look. Your partner is telling you that you're beautiful, and he whispers all the things he loves about you in bed. Take his word for it.

Believe that you are someone who is sexual. Open your heart and your mind to your lover. Having sex is a *pleasure,* and if you embrace it, it can heal your mind, body, and soul. Overcoming your shyness can only happen when you are willing to release your inhibitions and allow yourself to discover what makes you feel like the amazing, sexual being that you are.

Eliminating Perfectionism

Better sex happens when you learn to relinquish control. When you stop trying to control everything and stop thinking that it needs to be "perfect" otherwise your lover is going to think you're terrible, that's when you set yourself mentally and physically free. That means you're going to have to give up the need to be perfect. Having *perfect sex* does not exist. When two people come together in that way, you can't dictate what's going to happen or how their bodies are going to react and respond. Sex is not something you can meticulously plan in detail every step of the way. It is an experience you're going to have to surrender to and see where to moment takes you and your lover.

What is a perfectionist? Well, they're an individual who has strong beliefs about the way things should go. The problem is that what they seek, which is perfection, does not exist in this world. The perfectionist then follows something he cannot get. The perfectionist is frozen by their inability to achieve their own lofty standard. According to some psychologists, the antidote is to question, analyze one's beliefs and replace these beliefs with more rational ones. They find it hard to be happy when things don't go their way, even getting distressed about it. Do you relate to any of the examples above? Then you might be a perfectionist.

Perfectionists can set unreachable goals for themselves sometimes, and then it hits them hard if they fail to accomplish those goals because of that high level of expectation they set for themselves. Aiming too high, especially when the expectations are unrealistic, is a surefire way to set yourself up for failure, even in the bedroom. When you spend far too much time planning for perfection, you come up with all sorts of excuses to procrastinate and delay your plan because it will never be perfect enough to be executed in time.

Here's something you might not be aware of. *Perfectionism is killing your relationship.* Think you are feeling pressured to be the perfect lover? Your partner feels just as pressured, too, if not more. When you hold onto the need to be perfect, you're projecting that pressure onto your partner, whether you realize it or not. They'll feel pressured to live up to your expectations and then feel guilty when they can't. That's going to put considerable strain on the relationship, and when that kind of tension exists, it's hard to feel close to each other the way. Instead of bonding you as a couple, every sexual encounter is going to drive an even bigger wedge between you. You'll feel upset that things didn't go the way you had perfectly planned it to in your head, and they'll feel upset thinking that they've let you down even when they tried.

Listen up, perfectionist. You're obsessing over *nothing.* Part of what makes sex so exciting is the unpredictability. You never know what each episode is going to bring, and that's part of the thrill. If you knew with certainty every time how your partner is going to perform or the way they were going to react, how long do you think it's going to be before that gets boring real quick? Sex that becomes too routine is not great for the relationship either.

Still not convinced that you might be a secret perfectionist where sex is concerned? Look at these indicators below and see how many you relate to:

- Your sex life is getting worse instead of getting better the way you thought it would.
- Meditation does nothing to help calm your mind and teach you the art of letting things go (perfectionists have a hard time letting go of anything).
- You notice that your partner is starting to avoid you and make excuses not to have sex with you.
- You're becoming even more critical than ever each time you look at your body in the mirror. What's worse, you're becoming unfairly critical of your partner's body too.
- You feel depressed at the idea that your sex life is not going according to plan.

- You start developing anxiety whenever you think about sex and what else you can do to make it "perfect." Not better, but *perfect.*
- You have no sense of humor when anything goes wrong. Even when your partner can see the funny side of the situation, all you can focus on is how badly it turned out because it was not what you wanted it to be. A couple who cannot laugh together is a couple who is not going to survive for very long.
- Every mistake to you feels like a catastrophe, even when it may be minor in reality.

The need for perfectionism is a confidence killer. When the woman is with a man who is a perfectionist, this spells disaster for the relationship. This trait is going to destroy the woman's confidence as a lover, and when that happens, any hope of having amazing sex is now non-existent. Perfect sex does not exist, and holding onto that need for perfectionism is doing your relationship more harm than good. To eliminate the need for perfectionism, this is what you're going to have to do:

- **Change Your Entire Outlook -** You need to do a complete makeover of your outlook when it comes to dating and sex. If you're hoping for everything to go perfectly all the time, the only thing you're going to end up with is a lot of disappointment. At the end of the day, it is not the end of the world if nothing goes according to plan. What matters most is the moment that you share with this person that you love or care very deeply for. This is a special time for the two of you to connect intimately, and if you're too busy harping on how the little details are not as perfect as they should be, you're going to miss out on an incredible bonding opportunity.

- **You're Good Enough -** The desire for perfectionism often stems from deep-seated insecurity. A belief that we may not be good enough as we are, which is why we strive to be perfect. We labor under a false misconception that our partners might leave us and find someone better if we fail to live up to their expectations. Here's the truth: *nobody is perfect.* There's not a single person walking around out there in the world today who can confidently say they are perfect and without flaws. You have a lot to offer, and if your partner still refuses to see all of that and only chooses to focus on your shortcomings, then they may not be the right person for you.

- **See Things as They Are -** In other words, be realistic. Sometimes you just need to look at things realistically, see the facts in front of you and accept that nothing can ever be as perfect as you want 100% of the time. There is only so much that you can control in life, and everything doesn't have to be perfect every single time. The road to mind-blowing, passionate sex is not always smooth, paved-out pathway, and sometimes you need to take a few hard knocks, bumps and stumbles along the way, but that's okay as long as you reach the destination in the end.

- **Learn to Take Chances -** Step outside your comfort zone. You never know where it's going to lead you to. Eliminate the need to be perfect and take away all that pressure you've put on yourself unnecessarily to be the best lover in bed. Sometimes you just need to relinquish control and say, *"what's the worst thing that could happen?"* Maybe the spur of the moment sex position you decided to take a chance on in the heat of the moment could turn out to be even better than anything you could have planned or imagined.

- **Learn to Compromise -** If you couldn't have everything done your way, ask yourself what would be the middle point that you would be happy settling on. At this stage, it is important to talk to your partner about what you're thinking and reassure them that you're working on overcoming this need to be perfect. Let them know it has nothing to do with them, and it is an issue that you're trying to work through. Tell them you appreciate their support as you try to make it better, and in the meantime, if they could work with you to find common ground and compromise, that would be extremely helpful. You might not want to bring up this subject, but it is vital for your relationship that they are on the same page and can understand where you're coming from. Adding assumptions and miscommunication to the already existing tension created by perfectionism is only going to make things worse a lot quicker.

Chapter 5: Foreplay Is Essential

After having sex with the same person for a long time, it can start to feel too routine and predictable. While there's nothing necessarily wrong with that, it can't be denied either that shaking things up certainly adds some spice into your love life. Otherwise, it's easy to predict what's coming next. You kiss, maybe cuddle and fondle a little, a few minutes of oral, have sex, and then it's done. When a couple starts to become too comfortable with each other, there's a tendency to become too complacent or lazy. Especially when it comes to foreplay. The effort that goes into seducing each other begins to dwindle.

For a woman, foreplay matters. Her lover needs to inspire her to have sex since women are not ready to go at the drop of a hat the way men are. Men enjoy foreplay, too, but it holds greater importance for women since she'll find it difficult to orgasm when she isn't fully aroused. What a lot of couples fail to consider is when the foreplay goes stale, so does the intimacy. Foreplay is the unsung hero, and it does not get the time or attention that it should. A study published by the *Journal of Sexual Research* indicated that men and women find 20-minutes of foreplay to be the ideal duration. However, results from the study shed light on the fact that most couples in the study reported only spending half that time on foreplay. This neglect was potentially the reason a lot of couples did not feel as satisfied as they could have been.

Making Foreplay Meaningful

When you care deeply about the person that you are with, that's when foreplay becomes a meaningful exercising in strengthening the intimate bond that only two lovers can share. It loses all meaning if you do it just because it is expected of you. Foreplay is often treated as the prelude to the big finale, and the important role it plays in bringing two people together is underrated.

That desire to want to pleasure your partner must exist, or foreplay is always going to be treated as an afterthought. Couples need to use the love and care they have for each other as a reason to want to keep their partners in a state of sexual bliss.

Good foreplay ensures that men get an erection and the women get the lubrication they need. Lovemaking is not about the sex alone, and skipping out on this very crucial step means you're missing out on what is probably one of the best parts about having sex. Men who complain about not being able to make their lovers orgasm could benefit from spending a little more time engaged in this exercise. Women need more time to get in the mood, and when she is not, it is unfair to put that expectation on her to climax when you do.

True, she may not have needed as much foreplay when you were first going out since you couldn't keep your hands off each other. But once the "honeymoon phase" is over, she's not going to be so quick to jump your bones. The more comfortable you become together, the more stimulation she may need before she's ready for an intense and satisfying lovemaking session.

A Woman's Guide to Better Oral Sex

Kissing, hugging, and fondling is only scratching the surface of oral sex. There are so many layers left to be explored, and you're missing out on a lot when you only focus on going down south as soon as possible and get to your orgasm. A woman's body is a soft, beautiful, and sensual thing, and you need to spend time worshipping it the way it deserves and show her how attracted to her you are. This way, she won't conclude that you're only interested in sex, and all you want to do is get right down to business and get it over with.

A man is ready for sex pretty much as soon as he hits the sheets or catches sight of your glorious naked body. He won't be thinking about prolonged foreplay *unless you actively try to prolong it.* A woman can help her man get better at oral sex by encouraging the following:

- Begin the foreplay even before you get to the bedroom and keep it going as long as possible by kissing and cuddling each other. A man will be eager to get to action once you're in bed together, and staving him off by delaying that moment ensures more time is spent building the intimacy through kisses and caresses.

- Before cunnilingus, ask your man to tease you by kissing you through your panties. Ask him to tease you, kiss you, and suck on you through the delicate fabric of your underwear until he is itching to rip it off to get to the real thing. If you want to keep teasing him to prolong the foreplay, cheekily tell him he can't take off your panties until he has you panting, breathing hard and begging for him to yank it off and kiss you there already.

- Stroke his penis through the material of his jeans or pants in slow, deliberate moves. Tell him how turned on you are feeling the bulge in his pants. As he gets harder with each stroke of your hand, pull his head close to you with your other hand and deepen your kisses, whispering in between how hard he feels.

- During cunnilingus, *tell your man what you want.* He's not a mind reader and unless you guide him and show him exactly how you can be pleasured, he's going to do it based on his experience of what he thinks works best. He's not going to spend very long down there too *unless* you tell him what to do. This direct instruction is going to be sexy because it shows him you know what you want and you're not afraid to ask for it, and it lets him know he's doing all the right things when you're begging him to keep going and don't stop.

- The more turned on a woman gets during foreplay, the more pressure and intensity she craves. Let the touching and kissing start soft and slow in the beginning and then increase the pressure by squeezing or gripping your partner's arms, legs, shoulders, or waist tighter. When he feels your getting more intense, he will be quick to reciprocate and his kisses and touches will grow intense too. Drive him wild by giving encouragement along the way as you tell him to kiss you harder and pull his head closer. Tell him how good it feels when he's massaging your breasts and teasing your nipples with his fingers. When he can see how visibly aroused you are, he'll want to keep going just to increase your pleasure.

- Touching yourself in front of your man will have his eyes popping out of his head. He'll be so mesmerized by the sight of you pleasuring yourself right in front of him he won't be able to tear his eyes away from you. Do this for several minutes, and then ask him to take over once you see him practically drooling over you. He'll be more than willing to let his tongue and fingers roam all over your body to replicate that pleasure.

- Guide his hands where you want them to go. Most men are turned on by a woman who takes control like this, and again he's going to appreciate some direct instruction. A man wants to know that they can please their lover and be great in bed. Help him out in this department by guiding him directly towards where your pleasure spots are. Grasps his hands and glide it along your entire body, from your neck and right down to your breasts and vagina. Every now and then, bring his fingers up to your mouth and suck on them when he least expects it.

A Man's Guide to Better Oral Sex

When done correctly, the buildup to set can be even more enjoyable than the act of sex itself. Especially when a woman knows how to tease her man and drive him crazy right before they get down to business. Men find their women seductive. Otherwise, they would not be trying to have sex with you. A woman who knows her way around a man's body is like a goddess, but now all women are going to be experienced enough to know right away which points of a man's body to stimulate in the right way so foreplay is long and passionate. The same way men benefit from a little prompting and guidance along the way, the woman does too. Savor the exquisite moment of being together and guide your lover towards prolonging foreplay by:

- Asking her to massage your scalp after a long, hard day at the office. The scalp is the doorway to make other sexual spot stimulations, and if you like a good head massage, make it a part of your foreplay routine. Relish in the way he ringers move gently with the right applied pressure in slow, circular motions. Verbalize your pleasure by moaning, letting her know what a good job she's doing so she'll keep going at it.

- Slowly move the massage to other areas of your body. Ask her to glide her fingers down from your scalp to your neck and shoulders. Let her take her time feeling your strong muscles under her fingers. Even better, turn around and face her when she's doing this, so she's massaging your shoulders from the front. Look into her eyes as she's massaging you slowly to add the intensity.

- When you're kissing each other, hold her hands and gently glide them across your thighs, hovering close to your erection. This move teases you and your lover. She gets aroused, feeling the hardness of your erection, and your longing for her increases as you try to restrain yourself from whisking her into the bedroom right then and there.

- Cup one hand under her chin and tilt her face towards you so you can look deep into her eyes. While maintaining eye contact, tell her in a deep, low voice that you want her to undress you with her eyes. Many women will be taken aback by this since it's not a request they hear very often. There's a good chance she's going to find this an incredibly sexy request, and as she begins undressing you, her arousal starts to spike. Eye contact is extremely erotic, and it adds an extra layer of passion into the mix. Reciprocate by undressing *her* with your eyes too.

- Ask her for a striptease. The sight of your skimpily clad lover moving in a provocative way in front of you as you use every ounce of willpower you have left not to jump her bones right then and there is enough to supercharge your arousal. Even better when you're doing this with someone you're in love with. Ask her to put on one of the sexy lingerie she owns (pic one that is your favorite), get some sensual music going in the background, and let the striptease commence.

- Get her to tease you as you kiss by licking on your earlobes every now and then. Ask her to gently blow on them, nibble, lick, or suck on them to heighten your stimulation. The earlobes are the most underrated erogenous zones of the human body, and it doesn't get enough time in the spotlight. Until now, that is.

- When your lover tells you how she likes it done when you go down on her, return the favor by guiding her towards a blowjob that is going to blow your mind. Tell her how hard you want her to suck you and how to tantalize the tip of your penis with her tongue. Like you, women benefit from knowing *exactly* what works.

When she knows she's doing a good job, she's going to give it her all.

- Talking dirty during foreplay is enough to drive any man crazy. During this stage, get your lover to tell you all the things she wants you to do to her. Or what she wants to do to you. Depending on the way you like it, tell her what kind of dirty talk gets your engines fired up. Tell her what you want to do to her, too, and let your eyes roam her body as you lick your lips to signal your lust for her. A woman telling you all the naughty, kinky things she wants you to do to her body while at the same time holding you back and telling you to stop will get you so riled up you'll be ready to make love to her all night long if you could.

More Ways to Enhance Your Oral Game

Oral sex is not a competition to see who can do it better. It's a time for lovers to worship each other's bodies in ways that don't involve intercourse. To explore every inch of this body, you love by experimenting with new techniques. Mixing things up regularly will never leave you feeling like you're stuck in a rut, even if you've been in a relationship for a few years:

- **Narrate It -** Alternate when your mouth is not busy pleasuring your partner's body by telling them *what* you're doing and *how.* Narrate what you're about to do, but hold back for a few minutes as you let them stew in their anticipation.

- **Be Creative -** Blowjobs don't have to always be done on the knees, and cunnilingus does not have to be only when you're in the missionary position. The beauty of sex is there are a lot of positions for you to play around it. Try it from different angles, change your body positions (depending on your flexibility). Don't be afraid to get creative.

- **Be Spontaneous -** Live in the moment, you don't need to schedule your oral sex time and routine. Whenever you're alone together and you randomly feel horny, turn an ordinary Netflix movie night into a quickie oral session (assuming your partner is up for it too, of course). Taking him or her by surprise is part of keeping the excitement alive. Unpredictability keeps you on your toes.

- **Get Help -** In the form of sex toys. Sex toys shouldn't be limited to solo acts of self-pleasure. They have a lot more potential than that, as you will soon quickly discover once you start incorporating them into your foreplay routine. Sex toys up the ante, so to speak, and your partner will get off on watching you contort with pleasure as they use these sex toys on you.

- **Use Your Breath -** Have you ever tried using your breath, hot and steamy after some foreplay, to stimulate your lover's nerve endings and heighten the intensity they feel? The next time you go down on the, stop to blow your hot breath on their sensitive nether regions and they'll be begging for your lips to make contact.

- **Don't Hold Back -** If you knew that you were making your partner moan loudly as the intensity of their sexual pleasure starts to build during foreplay, wouldn't you want to keep it going for longer? Don't hold back the pleasure you feel. Vocalize it, moan it, scream it, let your lover know what they are doing to you and how much pleasure they are inflicting on you. Show your partner that you're having a good time during foreplay, and they'll want to keep the good times going as long as possible.

Chapter 6: Making Better Sex – Creative Lovemaking Positions Going Towards Ecstasy

Couples with great rhythm always have great sex. When the chemistry between two people is that good, it's inevitable. Whether they're kissing, cuddling, or shaking the entire bed with the force of their lovemaking, rhythm is essential to the earth-shattering orgasmic sex that every couple longs for. When you're with a partner for the first time, things may start off a little awkwardly, but the first few kisses will usually be a good indication of what's coming.

What Makes It Better?

In a word? *Chemistry.* The all-important sexual chemistry is the key to great lovemaking, and it is a large part of what defines the rhythm a couple has together. Being sexually attracted to your partner at the start is important, of course, but what sustains the passion later beyond her sexy butt or his hot body is the *chemistry.*

Plato came up with a theory 2,500 years ago about sexual chemistry and love. The idea of the "twin-soul theory" was born from the notion that each one of us has another half of our soul out there in the world. Deep within us, there is a desire to be reunited with this soul. Plato's theory states the following:

".......a certain degree of our internal happiness and balance needs to be achieved and nurtured first. Only then, when we are reunited, does the essence of one person flow into the essence of another. This creates completeness, and there is no effort involved....". Thus, the term "soul mate."

When there is chemistry, the lovemaking is incredible. There's an unspoken awareness about the other, an understanding that does not need words to describe. The couple can *feel* the way they complete each other. It could be a one-night stand or a long-term relationship, either way, when there is chemistry, the sex is going to be amazing.

Chemistry and compatibility are not to be mistaken for each other. Compatibility is focused on the act of sex itself and not the attraction. Finding a partner who is compatible in bed is easier than finding one you have chemistry with. Chemistry is the cornerstone that determines the health and success of a relationship. If it's going to last, there needs to be chemistry. The perfect rhythm in bed is the byproduct of compatibility. Like music or dance, the rhythm you have together should be graceful, beautiful, with crescendos and decrescendos that flow so naturally.

Having great sex does not need a lot of switching between humping like a rabbit or thrusting your partner with slow, deliberate movements. Amazing, incredible, wondrous sex happens when you're someone who has both compatibility and chemistry.

Understanding A Man's Rhythm Control

A man is not going to be great in bed when he can't control his rhythm. Many men, especially when they're still young and inexperienced, attempt to emulate the frenzied thrusting and pumping movements they see in porn. No wonder they ejaculated faster than a woman can count to 10. What they should be doing instead is building up the momentum and rhythm slowly. Start off the lovemaking nice and slow, and let the pleasure build itself up gradually, culminating the wild thrusting when she's finally ready to be pushed over the edge and right to her orgasm. A man who is *truly* masterful in bed will always keep his lover guessing, never knowing what surprise move he's going to pull next.

The best advice couples can give themselves is to forget what porn movies do. If she always knows what you're going to do next, the sex is going to get stale pretty quickly. Great rhythm control is a combination of the following techniques:

- Begin with slow and steady motions before gradually increasing your speed. Make her believe you're about to orgasm, and then pull back, slow it down, and grind your hips to stimulate her clitoris.

- Once you've calmed down, gradually pick up speed again and repeat the motion. When she believes you're going to come again, throw her off track by slowing down once more.

- Shift your speed between slow and fast and back to slow again. This will allow both of you to prolong the lovemaking. It keeps her guessing too, and she'll be amazed at how long you can last in bed with great rhythm control.

At the end of the day, great sex comes down to you. Experiment with a few techniques and don't be afraid to take your time. Lovemaking is not a process that should be rushed. Instead, savor each moment, relish in the feeling of being connected as one with your lover. Surprise her, tantalize and tease each other, bring her to her orgasm and then pull back, keep her guessing. A man who keeps things exciting and lasts longer than she expects is a man she won't be able to resist.

Sex Techniques That Heighten Your Lovemaking

Making love is an art that is perfected with practice. As you become sexually savvy, you begin to wonder if there are any positions that can enrich your lovemaking and heighten the pleasure that you feel. In short, you're on the lookout for lovemaking positions that hold the promise of leading towards ecstasy, like the following positions below:

Fingering Her

The woman's entire vulva is a very sensitive area. To make her orgasm, you will need to massage the entire area around the vulva. Massage her all over except at the clitoris area.

Keep this motion going as you continue to ignore the clitoral area as long as you can. Massage the entire area around her vulva is going to heighten the sensitivity of the area. Keeping going for about a minute or two. Once she's stimulated enough, massage the area around her clitoris in a circular motion once she's wet enough. Experiment between wide circular motions, diagonal, up and down, big circles, smaller circles, mix it up. Experiment with different pressure too, starting slow at first before gradually increasing the pressure. Listen to the noises that she makes. You'll know when she is aroused enough. Once you feel her arousal building, increase your pressure and speed until she gets louder and you feel her body start to tremble.

The All-Access Position

This one will be sure to make her orgasm as you begin by kneeling between her legs, straddling her left leg as she lies on her side. Her right leg will be bent around your waist, a position that will allow you to fully access her vagina for maximum pleasure. The deeper penetration you get with this move will allow you to control your rhythm as you explore her body. To bring her to the brink of ecstasy, stimulate her clitoris as you thrust.

The Crab Position

There will be quite a bit of communication going on in this position to get it right. Start facing each other, and then the woman will slowly lower herself and put her legs on her partner's shoulders. She will be straddling her partner with her legs on either side of his body as she opens them as wide as she can. The woman will then bend her back so it's arched to the perfect angle and then throw her head back and enjoy the rhythm as she moves together with her lover.

The Leg and Shoulder Position

Hold her legs when she's on her back and drape it over your shoulders. Her body should be approximately at a 90-degree angle when you do this. Her legs must be on your shoulders to get the deep, vaginal penetration needed. Once she's moaning with pleasure as she feels you deep inside her, take her by surprise by grabbing onto her butt and lifting her pelvis slightly so it's tilted towards you. A small tweak in the position is all it takes for her to orgasm in mere minutes.

The Cradle Position

Another ecstasy-inducing position is *The Cradle*, where the woman will once be on top. This position provides the ultimate deep penetration that is sure to make her shudder. The man will position himself on a flat surface, legs in front. Lean back against a wall for support. The woman will lower herself onto the man, with her legs spread. He will grab her thighs and lift her up, bringing her down entirely on his shaft. Once she has reached around and held onto her lover for support, the man can go to town and thrust her until he brings her to the edge.

The Happy Baby Pose (Advanced Anal Sex)

This is the ideal position to penetrate her anally while you stimulate her clitoris with your fingers and have her writhing under you with pleasure. The woman should be on her back for this one, with her legs bent in the air. Her legs should be slightly shoulder-width apart, dripping her toes on both feet with her hands. This position allows for both vaginal and anal penetration, and you could surprise her by switching between both. When she's close to her orgasm vaginally, remove your penis and penetrate her anally, prolonger the pleasure she feels before you thrust into her vagina once more. Bring her to the brink a few times, pull back, and repeat. When you're ready to finish her, stimulate her clitoris as you thrust deep into her and she'll be moaning in ecstasy as her body climaxes.

The Lying Down Anal

This position allows both partners to relax enough so there's easy access to that area of the woman's body. She will begin by lying down on her stomach, with her legs flat against the bed. Her head will be turned slightly to one side while the man props himself above her on his arms. The man's legs should be straddling her on either side as he prepares to enter her, keeping his arms pressed over her to help her stay calm. Listen to the way she responds and let your rhythm develop gradually.

The Child's Pose

Have her sit back on her heels and lean forward, extending her hands in front of her while keeping her back straight. This position will make her feel good as she elongates her back muscles, and even better once you start thrusting her from behind. Being relaxed makes it easier to orgasm, and if the bed happens to have a bedframe, have her grip it while you hold onto her hips or butt, penetrating her even deeper.

The G-Spot Target

Have her position herself on the edge of the bed on all fours, like you're about to do the doggy style. You'll be standing behind her, gripping her hips as she arches her back towards you. Her butt will be lifted upwards when she does this. Position your legs outside hers, and then use your thighs to squeeze her knees, pushing them closer together. This move will tighten the way her vagina feels around your penis, an ideal position for G-spot stimulation.

The Bad Doggy

When either partner is on the brink of an orgasm, switch it up and surprise your lover by going with the *Bad Doggy* position. Both couples will experience the climactic edge that we all want to achieve in sex, taking the regular *Doggy Style* position up a notch. The woman will be on her knees, resting against the edge of the bed or the couch (depending on which one she finds more comfortable). Her hips will be spread wide as she leans forward, bracing herself as her partner plunges into her from behind. With both hands gripping either side of her butt, the man is free to go as wild with his thrusting as he likes. Each time she moans louder, plunge into her a little deeper and harder.

The Vaginal Intensity

Position her face down on the bed. Her knees should be slightly bent under her so her hips will be raised upwards. For better comfort, positioning a pillow under her lower abs will help if she needs it. Tower over her, propping your weight on your arms and then thrust into her from behind. This position will make her vagina feel snug around your penis, making you feel a lot bigger inside her. The deep penetration in this position will have her crying out with pleasure at how good it feels. Switch between shallow thrusts and deep breaths to last longer.

The Perfumed-Garden Positon

A combination of chemistry and compatibility can make lovers feel so in tune with each other it is almost as if time stops in its tracks. This position is going to make the woman feel pleasure so great her back is going to arch in response. She starts by lying on her back with her legs in the air. Her lover will grab her hands so he can look deep into her eyes as he is drilling into her, using his hands to stabilize himself with each thrust. There's something erotically mesmerizing about looking deep into your lover's eyes as you channel the love you have for each other back and forth without words. Just moaning and panting that give away how good it seels to be connected as one.

Go the Extra Thrust and Switch Your Strokes

Once a couple is in the penetration stage of their vigorous lovemaking session, there's a technique a man can do to thrust even deeper into his lover and completely surprise her, just when she thought he couldn't get any deeper. The best position to pull this off would be anytime a woman has her legs spread while her hips are elevated ever so slightly. Once the man is inside her as deep as he can get, pause for a brief second and then thrust a little more before pulling back. Begin slowly at first until you've built a steady rhythm and then move faster and faster keeping pace with her panting and moaning. A little push can go a long way in intensifying the pleasure for both partners.

Pounding your lover like a jackrabbit will only guarantee that the man gets his orgasm quickly even before the woman has had a chance to get close to hers. Once you've mastered the deep push, intensify the pleasure *even more* by switching your strokes:

- **Slow and Short -** Give your lover the stimulation of her life with slow and short stroke than gently massages the sensitive opening of her vagina. Thrust slowly with short strokes and watch her moan beneath you as you do as you tease her with the tip of your penis before penetrating her fully.

- **Slow and Long -** As you do this, you will experience every ripple of your lover's vaginal walls against your hard shaft. Watch her face change to looks of pleasure as she feels you deep inside her, moving in long, slow, measured thrusts.

- **Fast and Short -** You'll do what you did with the short stroke, except this time with more speed. The rapid sensation will stimulate her vagina when you do this right before the full penetration.

- **Fast and Long -** You'll recognize this move as the jackrabbit maneuver a lot of younger men tend to do, copying what they saw in porn. It is a great position to bring in at the end as the deep thrusts and penetration are going to send her straight to her climax after all that initial teasing.

Chapter 7: Make Her Scream and Leave Him Breathless

The Big O is a concept that still seems to elude a lot of couples, especially the young novices who are only just beginning their foray into the world of sex for the first time. Some couples are not even *sure* whether they've had an orgasm or not, which only goes to show how little they know about the subject. Luckily, there's always room for improvement in all things sex. Men orgasm quickly while women need a bit more time is the general understanding most couples have, so it's no surprise that some are completely blown away by the fact that there are *several* types of orgasm a woman can experience. That's right. *Several.* There is even something called a nipple orgasm, something completely unheard of by most couples unless you've done your thorough research, or you're an expert on the subject.

Oh yes, women can have several kinds of orgasms and a lover that knows how to help her achieve all of these when they're making love is a sex god. Well, to her at least. Some men might find this felt overwhelming. It's hard enough to get a woman to come the usual way, let alone try to stimulate her in several ways to help her climax. Since they probably didn't even know this was possible, men might be awed and baffled at the same time. But fret not, it's not as difficult as it initially sounds. It's a matter of knowing how to stimulate her in the right spot, in the right way that will leave her with an earth-shattering orgasm as your name escapes her lips.

Sometimes an orgasm can be hard to come by when the body is so used to following the same old pattern. Which is probably why routine sex starts to get boring after a while. There is no excitement, no surprise, and when the body knows what to expect, the physical reaction is going to plateau eventually after you've been doing this for some time. The body needs to be kept on its toes, never knowing what to expect. The surprise is part of the overall thrill, and if you've ever had to catch your breath after your partner pulled a surprise move that left you panting and gasping, you'll know how important excitement is to keep the passion going.

The problem with orgasms is the way that we've been programmed to think about them. They are commonly thought of as nothing more than a means to an end. Something you "finish" your sexual encounter with. They are quite literally referred to as "climax," but does that mean they always have to be left for the grand finale? Not at all. The best kind of orgasm is the one that happens involuntarily, a culmination of the overall pleasure that has been building between you and your significant other. Couples don't spend enough time getting to know each other's bodies, learning what makes it tick. Sex is *not* all about the orgasms, and this is the kind of thinking that needs to change if you're hoping to experience more of them.

Before you experiment with any of the different techniques below, be sure that your lover is aroused enough and in the mood for sex before you begin. Another important point to be mindful of is *not to focus* on the orgasm or trying too hard to get her to come. Enjoy the moment, take your time, explore, learn, and above all else, cherish the intimate moment you're sharing, and the experience will be that much more pleasurable.

- **The Nipple Orgasm -** It's no secret by now that the woman's nipples are among the most sensitive erogenous zones in her body. Stimulating her breasts enough will send the energy flowing throughout her body and down to her clitoris, awakening the genital area. Regardless of the size of her breasts, the nipples are the most sensitive point and since men love already love playing with a woman's breasts anyway, the trick is to now do it long enough until she can climax. Take your time figuring out what triggers her arousal the most and listen to the way she responds for clues on what to do next. If you notice her breath start to quicken and she starts to pant and dig her fingers into your shoulders when you're teasing her nipples with your tongue, that's a cue to keep doing what you're doing.

- **The Clitoral Orgasm** - Most people would refer to this as a regular orgasm. When a woman's clitoris is well and truly stimulated intensely enough, it can lead to a short orgasmic peak. This usually lasts no more than 30-seconds or so. The woman's clit needs to be stimulated either directly or indirectly for her to achieve this, and a man can use his fingers, mouth, or a vibrator to do it. Once she has peaked through this technique, her clit becomes hypersensitive. Some women might even experience a little pain. The clitoris area can be stimulated either orally or through a couple of sex positions. While a clitoral orgasm does feel good, the pleasure felt here can't compare with what she experiences through vaginal orgasms.

- **The Vaginal Orgasm** - The bundle of nerves at the entrance of a woman's vagina makes it one of the more sensitive erogenous zones. Besides the clitoris, this is where most women experience the greatest pleasure that is soon followed by an orgasm (although not always). The entrance of the vagina is sharp and shallow, and the orgasm experience in this area might be sharp and explosive, like the kind experienced through clitoral orgasm too. It can feel extremely pleasurable to her when the man is penetrating the entrance of the vagina in shallow strokes, and as he moves deeper, the pleasure becomes even more intense.

- **The G-Spot Orgasm** - One of the most elusive areas for many couples is the G-spot of the woman's body. Most men have trouble even locating the G-spot, let alone attempting to give her an orgasm with it. The area is located inside the vagina on the upper wall under the pubic bone near the entrance. Inserting an index or middle finger into the vagina, curling, or hooking the finger towards her clitoris will lead you right to this spot. You'll know when you've arrived because this area is going to feel different from the other areas of her vaginal walls. It is a soft, ridged and fleshy hill that feels almost like a combination of a soft palate and a hard tongue. The area is also going to be swollen and engorged when she is aroused. Some women have their G-spot located near the entrance to the vagina while others have it further inside. All women have them and when stimulated enough, she will feel an overwhelming, intense pleasure unlike any of the other orgasms she experiences. It will be overwhelming, intense, and with the right partner, meaningful and she will be deeply satisfied and relaxed afterward.

- **The Anal Orgasm -** Despite their trepidation in the beginning, once a woman experiences an anal orgasm, there is no going back. Another little known erogenous zone of her body that is filled with sensitive nerves is the anus, and an orgasm in this area is rough, raw, physical and earthy. Not all women are going to be open to the idea of anal stimulation at first, so listen to your partner and respect her wishes. The orgasmic experience can be explosive when it happens and anal sex becomes easier when she is well and truly aroused. It is important to remember to use a lot of lube in this area to protect the sensitive tissue surrounding it.

- **The Cervical-Uterine Orgasm -** Tantric sex practitioners believe this to be probably the most meaningful, special, and profound type of orgasm that a woman can experience on a physical level. For a woman, her cervix is tied to her feminine core, where her heart, creativity, sense of self and entire wellbeing resides within this core. When she orgasms through this approach, it will be deeper and more intense than anything she has ever felt, even compared to the G-spot orgasm. With the right lover, it will be accompanied by intense feelings of love and a connection so deep that some women might cry because they feel so satisfied in every way. The experience of pleasure is so profound that it is indescribable. This is considered a whole-body orgasm, and when a woman experiences this, it is a day that she will never forget.

- **The Throat Orgasm -** Believe it or not, she's capable of achieving her orgasm while she's giving you a blowjob, especially when she's deep-throating you. This happens when her pituitary gland, located right at the back of the throat, is aroused enough, although the experience might also be due to the physiological side effect of holding her breath to suppress her gag reflex as she is taking you in. When she's giving you and oral and she's stimulated, large quantities of saliva and mucus are produced. These can be rather viscous and when the fluids are released, it is what some might consider an ejaculation of the throat. It can be a pleasant surprise for the woman to experience this while she's going down on you. Some women might have such a strong orgasm in this position that she has to stop giving you head for a while until she can catch her breath again. A common misconception is that women don't enjoy giving head or that they are merely doing it because their partner expects it. The truth is, women stand to benefit from this as much as men do, although she needs to be aroused quite a bit before this can happen.

How to Make Her Scream While You're Inside Her

Give your woman an explosive lovemaking session she will never forget the next time you're in bed together after reading this. It may be difficult for a lot of women to achieve the Big O through penetration, but it's not impossible, and here's how you do it:

- Kiss her. Kiss her softly, kiss her hard. Kiss her with deep passion because it's all about the intimate connection for her woman. Connect with her and her body will succumb to you.

- Cuddle her instead of straddling her right away. When you're spooning while you're thrusting, it's easier to stimulate the rest of her body and increase her arousal. Gently tug her hair if she likes to feel dominated, massage her breasts and use your fingers to tease her nipples until she's gripping her fingers into your back and shoulders, crying out with pleasure.

- Focus on every aspect of her body. Run your hands all over her body when you're on top of her and thrusting into her. Glide your hands from her neck, over her breasts and all over the beautiful, soft curves of her body. Spank her on her butt, lift her up, turn her over, change positions when she least expects it. Once your hand reaches her clit, rub it while you're still thrusting in and out of her. Start with light pressure at first and then increase it as she gets closer to her orgasm.

- If she's into it and so are you, dirty talk can add a little heat to your lovemaking session. A woman needs to feel desired. Do a good job of that and she's not going to orgasm once, but multiple times throughout the session. Tell her how soft and delicious her lips feel. Tell her how unbelievably nice and right she feels around your shaft.

- Let her know you're getting as much pleasure out of this as she is by vocalizing. Moan, pant, growl in her ear how sexy and beautiful you think she is. Make it clear that she's driving you insane with pleasure.

How to Make Him Breathless and Wanting You More

A man is happy anytime he gets to be in bed with a woman naked and having sex with her, but his pleasure can be intensified with the right lover who will give him an orgasm he is not going to forget anytime soon. The techniques below will be sure to leave him breathless and wanting more of you he can't wait to go again:

- **Do The 'Pop'** - Make your man's eyes roll back in his head when you're giving him fellatio by sliding your mouth wall the way down to the base of his penis. If you need to, use your hand as an extension, placing it at the base of his shaft. Once you reach the bottom, turn your mouth into a vacuum as you suck him hard and ever so slowly drag your mouth and lips all the way back up to the top again. Remember to go very, very, *very* slow, be deliberate about it. Once you reach the head, release the suction with a popping noise, look him cheekily in the eye, and then repeat from the beginning.

- **Right on Point -** The perineum is the most sensitive area for a man and is packed full of nerves just waiting to be stimulated. The perineum is the area that lies between his balls and his butt. Pleasure him here and you'll send him straight to orgasmic heaven. Get into the reverse cowgirl position (so he gets a glorious view of your behind too) and keep an eye on his balls. Once you see his testicles begin to rise (which means he is about to reach his climax), lick your fingers and then press his perineum and watch him cry out with pleasure.

- **Stimulate the Frenulum Too -** There's a small bump that can be found on the underside of the penis. It's easier to spot on a circumcised penis and this bump happens to be incredibly sensitive. If he has one, suck on his frenulum while you're stroking your penis with his hand during a blowjob and leave him panting for more.

- **Nice and Sloppy Does It -** Don't be afraid to get a little sloppy, because some men love this. Looking him in the eye, make a show of licking your palm slowly in front of him and then place your hand around his shaft to get it wet. Continue looking him in the eye as you spread your wet palm around his entire member before going down on him with your mouth. It'll drive him crazy.

- **The Triple Threat -** Send him straight to his sexual stratosphere by stimulating three specific pleasure points at the same time just as he is climaxing. Once you sense he's close to coming, cup his balls while simultaneously pressing on his perineum. Those two pleasure points and the third being him inside you will have him moaning your name and believing you're a goddess in bed.

- **Command Him -** Not in a bossy way, but a sexual one. Men love it when a woman is assertive in bed and knows what she wants. That is a turn-on for a lot of men, so tell him what to do, and you'll have him eating out of the palm of your hand. Once you sense he is close to the edge, look him dead in the eye with a seductive smile and tell him you can't wait to see him come right in front of you.

- **Sucking the Tip Through the Tits -** Apply a generous amount of lube over your breasts and lie down on your back. Press your breasts together and get your man to kneel right over you and thrust his penis between your cleavage. While he's doing this, gently suck and lick the tip of his penis to drive him absolutely insane with pleasure.

Chapter 8: It's Not Finished

Intercourse and foreplay are the most common thoughts that spring to mind when you think about sex. Most couples think that's all there is to it. Foreplay to get each other aroused, sex, and you're done. Not a lot of thought is given to what happens *after* sex. The post-coital play that is still very much part of the overall experience, but gets neglected too often. Did you ever stop to think you might be overlooking the *best part*? The emotional and physical intimacy that correlates your overall levels of satisfaction? Probably not, so let's talk about afterplay and why it matters.

Why Don't We Engage in Afterplay Enough?

For two possible reasons. One, we're tired after all that vigorous lovemaking. Two, we don't understand how important it is to bond with our partners after sex. In 1979, James Halpern and Mark A. Sherman co-wrote *Afterplay: The Key to Intimacy* in which

264 American women and men were observed as part of the research. In that study, the majority of the couples surveyed fell asleep within an hour after they had sex. The rest of the couples were reportedly dissatisfied with their afterplay experience. The participants who *did* enjoy post-coital afterplay agreed that it did correlate directly to the happiness they experienced in their relationship.

Afterplay helped the body cool down after sex, made the experience a lot more enjoyable, strengthened the bond the couples had, and promoted a healthy relationship dynamic. Engaging in afterplay led to more sex too, since the closer the couples felt to each other, the most they craved that intimacy.

It may not be the most exciting part of sex, but it is still an important aspect, nonetheless. We can't fault our partners entirely if they fall asleep after sex. It's the body's natural reaction to the parasympathetic nervous response that happens when the body experiences an orgasm. Sleep happens naturally when our bodies and minds feel deeply relaxed. After sex, a man's brain releases several chemicals into his body, including oxytocin, norepinephrine, vasopressin, serotonin, prolactin and nitric oxide once he has ejaculated. Prolactin, vasopressin, and oxytocin are the reason he feels drowsy and falls asleep after he has had an orgasm. For men, their heart rate and breathing return to normal once they've had an orgasm whereas a woman's body stays active a lot longer after she has had her orgasm. This is why she may be awake long after her partner has dozed off peacefully.

What Is Afterplay and What's Involved?

Anything that a couple does together immediately after they've had sex is considered afterplay. Most of the time, this involves either caressing, cuddling, talking, or all of it. Engaging in afterplay does not always have to entail more sex. Snuggling, taking a bath together, massaging each other, even hugging each other after sex is still considered afterplay.

More intercourse could happen if you're aroused enough, but that's not always necessary. If you've got the energy for it, by all means, why not. But the primary reason to engage in afterplay is to help each other work through those moments of vulnerability. The experience will usually last no more than a couple of minutes before the couple falls asleep or leave the bed to go and do something else. It is important for couples to engage in this after they've made love for one simple reason: *people are vulnerable after they've had sex.*

The love and affection that happens after sex has taken place is the key to improving and strengthening the intimacy and relationship. Even more so if the couple experiences any difficulty during sex. They may feel upset, uneasy, or plain uncomfortable after it's over. They're worried if they've let their partners down, maybe even feel embarrassed, worried, or afraid to talk about it. Those emotional and mental blocks can create an invisible barrier and the couple may pull away from each other emotionally and physically.

When a couple doesn't engage in post-coital intimacy, they're wasting a valuable bonding opportunity. What a couple should be doing instead of immediately rolling over and picking up their phones, falling asleep, or leaving the bed hurriedly to do something else is to stay in bed and stay close to each other. Cuddle, kiss, caress, whisper in your partner's ear and tell them how much you love them. Tell them everything you loved about being together a few moments ago and how connected you felt. Reassure them and see what a difference it makes in your love life.

If there are times when you feel that all you want to do is go to sleep and you're tired, that's okay. It happens sometimes, even between two people who love and care deeply about each other. Our bodies are not machines, after all, we do get tired after a long and busy day and a vigorous sex session that zapped any remaining energy we had left. Once in a while is not a problem, but where possible, a couple should try to make engaging in afterplay an important after-sex ritual.

Afterplay is Crucial and Here's Why

Post-coital depression is a very real condition. This happens when one or both partners feel unhappy after they've had sex. The feeling of "emptiness" inside them for reasons they may not always be able to explain can be aggravated if they feel neglected after sex. This is where afterplay comes in as an opportunity to help each other alleviate those feelings by spending a few quiet moments bonding together. Even if it is for only 5-minutes, it's better than not doing it at all.

No matter how long you've been together as a couple, you still need to work on strengthening your bond. Many couples get complacent after they've been in a relationship for a long time, and spending time strengthening and nurturing the connection they have falls by the wayside. Post-coital depression can be staved off when both partners try to reconnect after the physical and emotional experience they've just shared. A study conducted in 2014 even reinforced the fact that couples who spent time engaging in afterplay reported greater levels of sexual satisfaction.

A couple engages in erotic fantasies and role play when they're having sex together, taking on different personas in bed, dirty talking, doing things they may not normally do if they're feeling adventurous. Afterplay gives these couples an opportunity to step back after it's over and remind each other that they are there for each other. Women are particularly vulnerable and need to be reassured that their partners were interested in more than sex or that they were able to satisfy them in bed.

Afterplay is not just necessary, it's *vital* to the happiness of your relationship because:

- **It Cultivates A Healthier Relationship -** Afterplay that involves a lot of communication can have an immensely positive impact on the relationship. Since this is when couples are at their most vulnerable, they'll be a lot more likely to share their deepest, most intimate thoughts with their lovers which only brings them closer together as a couple.

- **Your Bond Grows Stronger -** Sure, you may bond in other ways when you're not having sex (spending time together, going on dates, etc.), but the bond that happens after sex is different. This is the time when couples are emotionally raw and vulnerable. A time when their guard is down and they bare their soul in a way they don't normally do. The cuddling, kissing and caressing that happens during this time brings you closer together mentally, emotionally and physically in a way that can't be replicated outside the bedroom.

- **It Gives Her Time to Cool Her Body Down** - Men can cool their bodies down within mere minutes, but women need a longer time to completely cool off after they've had sex. When a man's body has returned to normal, women are probably still craving some intimacy. Afterplay is a way to help her out and show her that you still care about her needs by showering her with intimacy until her body has had enough time to cool down and go back to normal too.

- **Sex Becomes More Enjoyable** - The University of Kansas carried out research into sexual behaviors and discovered that women find foreplay and afterplay more enjoyable than the actual intercourse. The study indicated that when a woman knows that the foreplay and afterplay are going to be enjoyable, she's likely to reciprocate more during intercourse, hence better sex every time.

- **It Paves the Way for More Sex -** Sometimes, massaging or kissing your partner, trailing your fingers along the curves of their bodies, and whispering how incredible you think they are can lead to another round of foreplay and sex. It's slow and sensuous, but it is effective in paving the way for longer sex marathons and multiple orgasms to take place.

How to Enhance Your Afterplay Sessions

For one thing, afterplay *should not* be used as an opportunity for you to conduct a postmortem on the sex you just had. If something was lacking or something made you uncomfortable, you should talk about it but at a later time. Don't bring up anything that might sound remotely negative or like criticism when your partner is at their most vulnerable state. There is a right time and place for everything, and a sexual postmortem is not on the agenda if you're looking for better afterplay sessions.

Afterplay *is not* the time you should be sharing your sexual grievances either. Obsessing about what you think went "wrong" or what "could have been better" is only going to make you and your partner feel worse about yourselves. What you should be talking about instead is everything that you enjoyed. Keep it light, playful, warm, and accepting so your partner feels comfortable enough to share what they loved about having sex with you that they otherwise feel shy talking about.

Other ways to enhance your afterplay experiences include:

- **Not Talking About Problems -** Discussing your issues is best left to another time, not when your partner is trying to bask in the warm and happy glow of the lovemaking you just had.

- **Tell Them How You Feel -** Pour your heart out to your partner. This is the best time to tell them everything you want them to know about the way you feel. Tell them you love them, how much they mean to you, how you would do anything for them, how your life has become so much better ever since they became a part of it. Talk about what you love about having sex with them, reinforce the love and care so they have no doubt in their mind that this relationship is built on more than just great sex alone.

- **Massage Each Other -** The intimate, skin-to-skin contact is a great bonding activity for both partners. Nothing like a good massage to induce feelings of deep relaxation and the sensual touch that takes place helps to strengthen the bond of intimacy and trust.

- **Kiss Each Other -** You did a lot of kissing while you were making love, but it was different. Those kisses were filled with fiery passion, lust, heat, and hormones. The kisses you share during afterplay, on the other hand, are warm, exuding love, slow, intimate, and unhurried. With every kiss you share, you're communicating without words what your partner means to you.

- **Take A Shower Together -** If you do want to leave the bed almost immediately, why not do it together and hit the shower at the same time. You got dirty together, and now it's time to get clean together. All the afterplay suggestions that have been discussed so far and be incorporated into this activity. When you're massaging the shampoo on each other's scalp or lathering soap all over your lover's bodies, massage them, kiss them, hold them close, talk to each other, laugh together.

Talking About Afterglow

Some couples experience a warm, happy, fuzzy feeling after they've had sex. There's a sense of contentment and satisfaction that still lingers long after the act of getting physical together has ended.

Researchers call this the "sexual afterglow", and they believe it helps to bring couples closer together romantically.

It's hard not to feel close to someone when you're feeling perfectly blissful and happiness seems to be coursing all through our body. One study by the *Association for Psychological Science* suggests that this lingering feeling of contentment is an indication of the quality of the relationship the couple has. The same study goes on to suggested that couples who bask in this ambiance for up to 48-hours after sex can strengthen the bond that they feel. This new body of research was compiled after scientists came together to pool the data they collected from two separate studies carried out on newlyweds.

The research involved 214 couples overall and took place over a span of two weeks. Every night, the couples had to journal whether they had sex or not. They also ha to rank their sexual and marital satisfaction using a 7-point scale. Researchers made notes about the couples' "marital quality" and "marital bliss" at the start of the study, and then again 4-6 months later. Here's what they found out: *Couples who experience an intense or stronger afterglow reported higher levels of sexual satisfaction as much as two days after they've had sex, and they were happier in the relationships they had over time too.* The couples in the study only had sex an average of four times throughout the 14-day study, which indicated that afterglow was strong enough to keep the satisfaction going even if they didn't hump like bunnies every day. However, the quality of their relationship was linked to the lingering contentment and happy satisfaction they felt thanks to the afterglow.

Yet another interesting finding that came out of the study was how men and women did not differ in the levels of sexual satisfaction they felt. When they did have sex, it came as no surprise that they reported greater levels of satisfaction that lasted not just on that day, but as much as 24 to 48-hours *after.* Researchers believed that the oxytocin and dopamine receptors of the brain are activated during sex, and these same neurochemicals are responsible for the romantic love that is felt between a couple. Essentially, afterglow serves to enhance the connection between a couple, pretty much the way afterplay does.

Sex is more than a means to satisfy your urges. As the studies have revealed, it is very much a bonding activity that can keep the relationship strong enough to withstand the test of time. Perhaps that's one of the reasons some couples don't fall apart so easily no matter what challenges and tests life puts them through. The strength of their relationship is enough to overcome it all.

What Afterglow Can Tell You About Your Relationship

Husbands and wives generally begin to experience diminishing marital satisfaction in the early months after getting married. But the longer the afterglow lingered, the greater the marital satisfaction they felt over time, according to what researchers discovered. When afterglow is present, it signals that the couple is satisfied with the relationship they have, although researchers did admit that more study was needed to gauge if the same findings could be applied to older couples who have been together a lot longer. The newlyweds in the earlier study were young, and further research could shed light on whether afterglow could be as impactful on older long-term relationship couples too.

For now, researchers can only hypothesize afterglow is a good indication of the strength of a relationship and possibly linked to less cheating, too if the couple had no reason to be dissatisfied enough to cheat. Besides keeping a couple strong, there's another purpose that afterglow serves too. It increases the likelihood of the couple conceiving. It turns out the odds increased in their favor two days after having sex, which is good news for couples who are actively trying for a baby. Looks like afterglow is beneficial from an evolutionary standpoint too.

Chapter 9: Spicing Up Your Sex Life

Wake up. Go to work. Come home. Exercise. Eat. Have sex. Sleep. Repeat. We're creatures of habit and routine. While that's not necessarily a bad thing, it can put your sex life at risk of becoming dull, mundane, and well, just plain *boring.*

Overcoming the Boredom

As much as we may love our partners, it has to be said that boredom does happen. When it hits, some couples may be tempted to go astray when they feel emotionally and sexually bored. By nature, humans are attracted to change. We need variety now and then to keep things exciting. Even when venturing out of our comfort zones is not something we seek out actively, a little excitement that shakes things up once in a while can make us feel alive again. When everything becomes too routine, boredom inevitably follows.

We choose to make that commitment and get into long-term relationships for several good reasons. We want the emotional security that comes with it, we want the happiness and sense of belonging that comes from sharing a special bond with another. Yet, at the same time, by committing to one relationship, we are also limiting our option. Could it be fair to say that boredom was perhaps inevitable? We're living longer, enjoying greater leisure, and we've got higher emotional and sexual expectations from our partners. These and a lot of other factors today make it unlikely that couples who stay together for decades will *never* experience boredom together.

For many couples, particularly the ones who believe in romanticized versions of love and marriage, disappointment, hurt, and sadness quickly follow when they realize their partner may be boredom with their sex life. The electrifying passion they once felt begins to wane over time. The sex starts to get too routine and mechanical. Some people feel unhappy and grieve over the loss of that aspect of their sex life, while others may stray. But there are couples who do something else entirely. They find *new* ways of keeping the excitement alive in their relationship. Yes, breathing life back into an old relationship is absolutely possible, but it does require that the couple work together to get it done. To rekindle the excitement, couples need to surprise each other in new and unexpected ways. Not just physically, but emotionally too. Introduce new ideas in the bedroom, try new positions, use sex toys, maybe even venture outside the bedroom to find the cure of sexual boredom. How? With *sex games,* stripteases and having sex in new places. Better yet if you could combine all three elements together.

Here are some ideas to help you get started:

Scenario 1: Going Away for the Weekend - If it's been a while since you went away for the weekend, this might be just what you need if things have been feeling a little lackluster lately. Take a break from your regular routine and head somewhere the two of you can be alone together. Once you arrive and settle in, it's time to head out to dinner. While your partner orders the meal, you slip away into the ladies room, take off your panties, and put them in your purse. Meanwhile, he has no idea as you make your way back to the table. The food comes, you're enjoying your meal, and then slowly slide your foot up to your partner's leg. He's surprised at first as your foot slides closer to his crotch, but then quickly reciprocates when he sees the cheeky smile you're giving him.

You slide closer as his hand travels up your leg, along the curve of your thigh until he gasps with surprise as he realized you haven't got your panties on. Whisper naughty things in his ear as his fingers begin to work their magic and when you finally feel so wet you're about to rip his clothes off, push your chair back, plant a kiss on his lips and tell him *"you know where to find me"* as you walk away seductively, swinging your hips to make sure he's got a good view of your butt as you make your way back to the room. He quickly pays for the dinners, rushes back the room, flings the door open, and is met with another happy surprise when you pull him close and push him on the bed. *"Sit there. I'm going to strip for you."*

The sexy music begins to play, you gyrate your hips slowly, turning around to make sure he can see every inch of you. You begin slowly undressing, watching his eyes grow wider and the hunger on his face becomes more apparent as you tease him with little glimpses of your flesh before letting it all drop to the floor and you're clad in nothing more than your bra and panties (which you put on again while waiting for him). Running your hands all over your body as you continue to sway to the music, move closer until you can grab him by his shirt, pull him up and whisper, *"Your turn."* By this stage, he's going to be so fired up with hormones the two of you are going to be in for a long night of lovemaking.

How to Climb Out of Your Sexual Rut

Love life feeling stale lately? That's a sign you're stuck in a sexual rut, and you'll need to work together to get out of it. It's okay to find yourself stuck; it happens even to the happiest couples. What matters is the way you work together to overcome it.

- **Talk to Each Other -** Communication is essential to overcoming this tricky stage of your relationship. But be mindful of *the way* you communicate. Avoid phrasing your words in such it way it seems like you're blaming them for the boredom you feel in the relationship. For example, don't say, *"We're stuck in a rut"* or *"The way the relationship is going right now is boring, don't you think?".* Instead, be gentle when you communicate and say *"Let's work together and figure out what we can do."*

- **Don't Get Angry With Each Other -** The first reaction by either partner might be to feel defensive but avoid getting angry with each other. It is important to communicate honestly, and you or your partner may not feel comfortable doing that if they know it's going to make the other person mad. Then again, if you *don't* talk about it, the problem is not going to fix itself, and acknowledging that there is a problem is the first step to repairing what might need to be fixed in your relationship. Getting angry or upset about it and lashing out at each other is only going to make the situation worse. Whenever there's a problem, especially something like this involving your sex life, stay calm, talk about it and try to work things out.

- **Try Some Nonsexual Changes -** The boredom you feel might not entirely be bedroom related. Perhaps your routine together has become too mundane in general. If you suspect that might be adding to it, try making some changes or do something new together. Try a new restaurant, go for a walk together, explore a new city, go away a short getaway together. A change of routine can feel refreshing if you've been doing the same old thing day in and day out.

- **Changing Your Look -** It's not a necessity, but if it makes you feel better and gives you a confidence boost, this is one to consider. Getting a makeover can make us feel like a new and improved version of ourselves, and a shift in perspective is enough to spark a sense of excitement again. Get a haircut, get some new clothes, new makeup, whatever you feel like to boost your spirits.

- **Keep Growing and Learning -** It's hard to feel bored when you're always learning something new and growing both as an individual and a couple. Even better, take up activities you can do together, so you're *both* learning, growing, and bonding at the same time. Pick up a new hobby, read a book together, take a new class or course, learn a new skill together. There's no end to the possibilities once you start looking and discovering something new you might not have known about each other can make you see your partner in a whole new light.

Scenario 3: Little Joyful Moments- Dealing with the everyday stresses of life can suck the joy we feel if we choose to let it happen. Planning little joyful moments that are both sexual and sensual can make you feel alive again and they don't always have to be grand, romantic gestures either. Plan a candlelight dinner together. Leave love notes in their purse. Send a sexy text in the middle of the day. Deliver flowers to your partner at work. Take a relaxing bubble bath together. Have breakfast in bed this weekend. Plan a trip next month. Surprise your partner with a gift if you know they've had a hard day. There's no end to the possibilities of what you can do to. Sometimes, alleviating the boredom could be as simple as bringing a smile to your partner's face again.

Scenario 2: Hotel Role Play - Treat your next hotel stay like a naughty sex adventure, and if you want to make it even more interesting, don't tell your partner what you're up to. Make the reservations (once you've confirmed they're free of course) but don't tell your partner what you've done. Invite them to meet you at the bar for a drink. Once you spot them sitting at the bar waiting for you, get the bartender to hand them a note and the key to the room (you would have given the bartender both in advance). Surprised, your partner opens the note and sees that you've written: *"You hold the key to an erotic evening you don't want to miss. I'll be waiting".*

Your partner makes their way up to the room, heart beating a little faster in anticipation and excitement, unsure of what awaits. When they arrive, they open the door and walk into the room, looking around at their surroundings. You come up from behind, hug, and kiss them as you whisper: *"I've been fantasizing about you all day."* You then begin to recreate a sexual fantasy you know they've been eager to try out, bringing to life as you watch their eyes grow wider with surprise and delight. Tease each other, play out your dirtiest, naughtiest fantasies all night long until you're both panting heavily and basking in the warm glow of post-coital bliss.

The Stripteasing Fantasy

Spicing up your sex life is not as hard as it may seem. It's a matter of figuring out what your partner likes, what turns them on and drives them wild and going for it! A little creativity with the right visual stimulation and you're going to have a hard time holding him back as he tries to ravage you. Any red-blooded male with a healthy sex drive is bound to have several fantasies at best running through his mind. One such alluring fantasy? *Stripteasing.* The expression in your eyes, the way your body sways to the rhythm of the music, the way you taunt him by running your hands all over your body while standing just outside of reach will make him yearn for you even more. He's bound to have fantasized about you several times, but seeing his stripteasing fantasy come to life with you as the star of the show? You'll probably have to tie him down to keep him from jumping you right there and then.

You don't have to be a sexy supermodel or a porn star to turn him on and make his wild fantasy come true. The secret to turning his striptease imagery into one that is better than anything he could visualize is to tease him *throughout* the day instead of doing it right before you jump into bed together:

- Sext him throughout the day and give him a taste of what's waiting for him when he comes home tonight. Focus on toying with his imagination, revealing just enough information, so he knows what's coming.

- Practice before your big debut. Learn some dance moves that focus on a lot of hip movement and swaying that will make it hard for him to tear his eyes away from you.

- There are only three rules to stripteasing you need to remember: *Tempt, Tease and Tantalize.* Move seductively in a way that accentuates the curves of your body, focusing on your breasts and buttocks but always tease him by staying out of reach. Close, but not close enough for him to touch. It will drive him crazy with longing for you.

- Take your stripteasing session up a notch with a pair of handcuffs or a silk scarf to tie him up. Restrict his movement and gyrate your body in front of him. If he tries to break free to grab onto you, wink seductively and tell him he's got to follow your rules. Tell him you're allowed to touch him, but *he can't touch you.* Keep gyrating your body in front of his face until he can't bear it any longer.

- Tease him by giving him a peek at the goods but no more than that. In between your dance moves and sashaying, pull your bra down so he can see a hint of a nipple. Sway your breasts in his face while you do this and then cover back up, giving him a cheeky wink as you do.

- Drop your inhibitions and lose yourself in the moment. You need to enjoy yourself as much as he enjoys watching you so your sexy dance doesn't look painfully awkward.

Other Ways to Turn Up the Heat on Your Sex Life

Sex games, role-playing and recreating fantasies can do wonders to revive the excitement you might have thought was lost in your relationship. The best part is most of the time; all you need is your imagination and some creativity. There's no end to the things you could try in the bedroom and when you're ready, let the creative, sexy time begin!

- Have sex while blindfolded and watch how your other sense comes alive. Every touch starts to feel electric and every sensation feels ten times more powerful.

- Watch porn together to bring you closer as a couple. We've all done it, *especially men,* so there's no point denying or trying to pretend like we don't. Instead of watching it solo, watch it together this time and see who gets turned on first.

- Put on a porn movie in the background and try to mimic what the couple on-screen are doing.

- Turn it into a sex game by challenging each other to see how many times a day you can have sex without repeating the same position twice.

- Go for another game where you and your lover try to do it in every room in the house and on every piece of furniture that can support you. See if you can get it done in a day, probably with an all-day sex marathon.

- Try having sex tonight using *all* the sex toys you have. Every single piece needs to be used at least once. No exceptions.

- Try dominating her in bed. 17% of women have reportedly tried bondage, and Durex's 2005 survey reported that at least 36% of adults in the United States have reportedly tried blindfolds, masks, and other bondage tools during sex. It's a huge part of the overall sexual fantasy aspect.

- Share your fantasies. Have each person write down five fantasies you would each like to role play or recreate, put them in a jar and take turns pulling one fantasy each out of the jar and get busy!

- Blindfold your partner and tease their body with different materials, textures, and sensations. Silk, feathers, whipped cream sprayed on their erogenous zones, anything you'd like as long as your partner is comfortable with it. Keep them gasping and guessing, wondering what's coming next.

- Indulge in a couple's erotic massage together if it's been a while since you've done that. Use scents that you both find relaxing and take turns helping each other relax. Make your movements nice and slow, appreciating the curves of your partner's body. Linger longer on the erogenous zones and listen to their moans as you sensually massage their sensitive areas.

Conclusion

Thank you for making it through to the end of *Better Sex*, let's hope it was informative and able to provide you with all of the tools you need to achieve your goals whatever they may be.

Mind-blowing sex. It is entirely possible, anywhere, anytime with the right partner and the right techniques. The basic rule of thumb to remember is to focus on stimulating your partner's senses and their bodies. This should be your primary focus, not the orgasm, and not the act of sex alone. Great sex is more than just a man and women being joined together at the genitals. It is about the chemistry, the rhythm, the compatibility, intimacy, bond and connection that they share that is unlike anything they have with anyone else. There's nothing quite like the feeling of two souls coming together as one and as the sex gets better, the relationship only grows stronger and the intimacy increases.

It is also about the way you approach sex too. You need to *believe* that you are a beautiful, sexual, erotic being. You need to *believe* that sex is a pleasure and not a dirty taboo secret that is not to be discussed. Forget everything that you have been programmed to believe. Toss all the myths, misconceptions and misgivings out the window. Better sex happens when you let go of the mental and physical chains that have been holding you back and devote your mind, body, and spirit to the experience. Devote yourself entirely to your lover as you give and receive love. Embrace this side of you; don't suppress it. Sex is a natural part of our human desire, and it is time we embraced that side of us and open our bodies and our minds to the immense possibility of greater, better sex.

Additionally, if you found this book useful and you are satisfied with it, you have the chance to delve deeper into the subject by purchasing other books from the same series:

- **Sex Positions**

A practical guide for beginners to play out your sexual fantasies for a better sex. Release your sexual energy and transform your sex life, Reach ecstasy for Men, Women and couples

- **How to Talk Dirty**

The complete sex book guide, examples to improve your sex life with new sexual energy. Drive your partner absolutely wild, become his sexual obsession and have the mind-blowing sex

- **Tantric Sex**

The complete guide to discover the best tantric secrets for meditation, yoga, massage and obtain a new sex life full of sexual energy. Tantra for man, woman, couples for a better sex

They are all part of the "**Sex life experiences**" series, available on Amazon in paperback, kindle or audio format.

Finally, I would be really grateful if you would like to write a review of this book and, if possible, help me by sharing it with your contacts. Your opinion is essential in order for me to offer you high quality work in the future.

CPSIA information can be obtained
at www.ICGtesting.com
Printed in the USA
LVHW080754081220
672143LV00036B/306

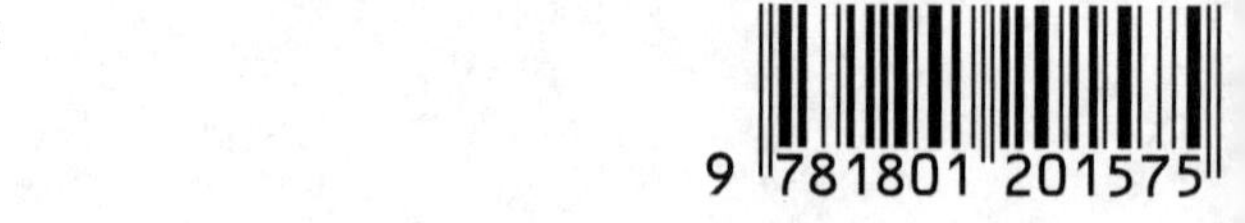